SOCIAL WORK

THE BASICS

Social Work: The Basics is an insightful introduction to the often misrepresented world of social work. Presenting a broad historical and contemporary view, this book dispels myths surrounding social work and explores its roots and its possible future. Questions covered include:

- How and why do people come into contact with social workers?
- What are the aims of social work – to help or to control?
- What is the relationship between social work and social policy?
- What is the role of the social worker?

Drawing examples from the full range of social work practice, this book is a valuable introduction for anyone beginning social work courses, considering a career in social work or with a professional or broad interest in social work.

Mark Doel is Emeritus Professor of Social Work at Sheffield Hallam University, UK. He has a wealth of experience in writing about, teaching and practising social work, having worked in the UK, USA, eastern Europe and Russia. He is the author of *Social Work Placements: A Traveller's Guide* (Routledge, 2010).

The Basics

SOCIAL WORK

THE BASICS

Mark Doel

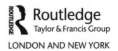

LONDON AND NEW YORK

First published 2012
by Routledge
2 Park Square, Milton Park, Abingdon, Oxon OX14 4RN

Simultaneously published in the USA and Canada
by Routledge
711 Third Avenue, New York, NY 10017

Routledge is an imprint of the Taylor & Francis Group, an informa business

British Library Cataloguing in Publication Data
A catalogue record for this book is available from the British Library

Library of Congress Cataloging in Publication Data
Doel, Mark.
Social work : the basics / Mark Doel.
p. cm. – (The basics)
1. Social service. 2. Social workers. 3. Social case work. I. Title.
HV40.D6333 2012
361.3 – dc23
2011049945

ISBN: 978-0-415-60398-0 (hbk)
ISBN: 978-0-415-60399-7 (pbk)
ISBN: 978-0-203-11423-0 (ebk)

Typeset in Bembo and Scala Sans
by Taylor & Francis Books

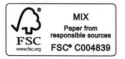

Printed and bound in Great Britain by the MPG Books Group

Dedicated to Jessica, Finley, Elsie and Shreya – the next, next generation

CONTENTS

ACKNOWLEDGEMENTS

It is not possible to name all the people who, over the years, have helped me to a fuller understanding of social work – all my colleagues, clients and students – but I do thank you all.

I received specific information and comments, for which I am very grateful, from Simon Cauvain, Kirsty Connor, Ann Davis, Brigitte Geissler-Piltz, Ruth Geuter, Anne Hollows, Valerie Hubbard, Paul Johnson, Tim Kelly, Jackie King-Owen, Vesna Leskosek, Pete Marsh, Tamsin McCullough, Pete Nelson, Jonathan Parker, Jonathan Scourfield, Ian Thomas, Janet Williams and Sandra Wilson. Sincere thanks to *Community Care* for various permissions and also for supplying an endless amount of helpful, current (at the time of writing) information. My sincere thanks to the Routledge team – Sophie Thomson, Andy Humphries, Rebecca Shillabeer, Nigel Hope and Emma Hudson – for their reliable encouragement through all stages of the book. Deepest thanks to Jan Doel for her forbearance in what was supposed to have been my first year of 'retirement'.

There was limited space for the Further Reading sections that conclude each chapter, and I would like to acknowledge the fact that there are many valuable readings that I have not been able to include, and to apologise to their authors for their absence.

PIONEER, INVESTIGATOR, AGITATOR
A BRIEF INTRODUCTION

One of the most interesting challenges in writing this book has been to decide how to slice up the social work cake, whilst not losing the sense of the whole (sometimes called a holistic perspective) that is so essential to social work. You will see from each of the chapter titles that I decided to use the major themes that illustrate the fact that people are not especially in agreement about what social work is. So, the book's structure reflects the contested nature of social work.

Does social work aim to reform the wobbly wheels of society or is it something much more radical, a fundamental challenge to the social status quo? Are social workers quietly heroic folk who do good and caring things; or are they controlling agents of the state, ready to whip your children away as soon as look at them? The people who use social work – are they *clients* with a professional and confidential relationship with their practitioners, *consumers* choosing this or that service like so many ice cream flavours, *experts* by virtue of their own experience, *claimants* exercising their rights or *users* of services? Is social work a noble calling or an everyday job, the newest profession or just another career in public service? Should the preparation of social workers be an education, an intellectual foundation in the social sciences and other humanities? Or is it a basic practical training to fit people with the competences to do specific tasks? And how tied to a particular time and location is it?

Is social work entirely defined by local context or are there universal elements that are everlasting and inalienable?

The very short answer to all these questions is yes. It is all of these things. These seeming opposites are in fact false dichotomies, examples of polarised thinking. All these facets are possible; indeed, all are an essential part of social work, creating their own tensions, as I hope each chapter will make clear.

Writing *The Social Worker* in 1920, Clement Attlee (then a social worker, later British Prime Minister) identified a number of roles for social workers. These included pioneer, investigator and agitator. For Attlee it is the social worker who sparks life into the ideas, plans and principles of the social theorist, the social reformer and the social revolutionary. Attlee optimistically declares that the pioneers of today are the prophets of tomorrow: yes, he is speaking of social workers. They add to the stock of social knowledge and investigate the consequences of social legislation; and 'every social worker is almost certain to be also an agitator', whether it is to battle against vested interests or to stir the apathy and complacency of the general public.

The view that social work should be partisan – committed to social justice and fighting for those who are oppressed – is just as relevant a century later. It might seem far removed from the desk-bound reality of some social work, but I have aimed in this book to describe what social work has been, what it is in its various current manifestations and what it can be. I hope it is a fair representation, but it is partisan – how could it be anything else yet stay true to social work?

The book contains many personal reflections and my hope is that these illuminate rather than obscure. The text inevitably reflects my own biography, as someone whose experience of social work spans four decades in the late twentieth and early twenty-first centuries, largely in England, but not exclusively. I have, therefore, been confronted by the conundrum of local and global that is the central theme of the last chapter. As I compose this introduction, a social work colleague writes from Palestine that 'social work students are required to do 60 hours per semester community work including donating blood to combat thalassaemia'. I smile at the response British social work students would be likely to have to this requirement. Yet, at the conclusion of their very different educations in Palestine and the UK, all will call themselves social workers, and rightly so.

There are many ideas in the book that have been written about elsewhere, and often in greater detail, but the style of the *Basics* series is not to reference within the text. No disrespect to the authors of these ideas is intended by the absence of direct reference. The Further Reading sections that conclude each chapter are designed to point readers to some of the significant texts and websites. Inevitably, there are many very good texts that it has not been possible to include.

I have some pessimism about the slide from professionalism to proceduralism in British social work, some comfort that social work is not singled out amongst professions for this treatment and that it is not a universal trend; and much optimism drawn from the enthusiasm of the social work students who will be the next generation of social workers, from the wisdom of the experienced social workers who teach them about social work in practical placements and from the alliances between service users and social work.

People with the least power and the weakest voices need social work, whichever society they live in. It is as important now as it ever has been that the wider public knows what social work is and what social workers do, and that they are agitated to support social work. I hope this book can contribute a little to this agitation.

Mark Doel
Sheffield, England
August 2011

1

REFORMIST OR RADICAL
SOCIAL WORK'S ROOTS AND DIFFERENT IDENTITIES

A social worker is expected to be both a firm footed realist and a clear eyed idealist.

F.P. Biestek, *The Casework Relationship*,
Chicago: Loyola University Press, 1957: 136

WHAT IS SOCIAL WORK?

At some point during the 1980s Margaret Thatcher, then British Prime Minister, was asked to comment on the problem of the growing ranks of the unemployed. She responded by declaring that they should do social work. The tale might be apocryphal but it contains the uncomfortable idea that social work is something that anyone can do, without any education or training. All that is needed is common sense, life experience and some time on your hands.

Qualified, experienced social workers were duly affronted by the Thatcher pronouncement and the suggestion that their work was so devalued. Yet, did this mean that there was no social work before the Certificate of Qualification in Social Work or its equivalent around the world? If we can speak about parents *teaching* their children and partners *nursing* each other, or communities *policing* themselves, why not embrace the notion of *social working* as something more universal than the work done by someone with a degree and a professional qualification?

This same phenomenon was described a century ago by Clement Attlee. He used the term 'social service' to describe every contribution that each member of society, individually or working through a group, brings to society. He notes that the Social Service movement of modern times (1920: 2)

> is not a movement concerned alone with the material, with housing and drains, clinics and feeding centres, gas and water, but is the expression of the desire for social justice, for freedom and beauty, and for the better apportionment of all the things that make up a good life.

He recognises that social workers have a very particular place in this general social service movement and that they are people who feel 'the claims of society' more than others.

Social work is a modern profession, but its roots stretch back into antiquity. The current professionalised form is one expression of social work that has developed as the result of social reformers, advances in knowledge and the rise of democratic ideas. The knowledge base and the skills have been formalised and continue to be developed and there is a distinctive training, a growing body of research and literature, a protected title and professional associations. Many of the values that underpin social work and the motivation that drives people to become a social worker are timeless and universal: from individual acts of charity to collective action that challenges injustice and oppression.

The scope of social work is daunting. In recent times social work services, in response to government policies, have tried to limit this scope through procedures to contain those who are eligible, but this has created its own additional work. Moreover, the joy of social work is its combination of the telescopic and the microscopic, its hard-to-define position and its unclear boundaries. The podiatrist works with feet, the plumber with pipes, but social workers work with the human and social condition.

DEFINITIONS

In the next few pages we will use definitions, metaphors and narrative stories to understand social work and how it is viewed.

The social work profession promotes social change, problem solving in human relationships and the empowerment and liberation of people to enhance well-being. Utilising theories of human behaviour and social systems, social work intervenes at the points where people interact with their environments. Principles of human rights and social justice are fundamental to social work.

International Federation of Social Workers, 2000,
modifying the 1982 definition

This example illustrates the limitations of definitions: first, in order to be succinct, they are framed at a general, abstract level. Fortunately, we have a whole book ahead of us in which to be more specific and illustrative. Second, where a definition does attempt to be definite, it is in danger of tying itself to time and place. The definition above replaced a 1982 version: is social work so time-specific that its definition changes in two decades? Does this definition of social work stand up in, say, rural China? We will explore these questions through the book and especially in Chapter 6.

More rounded than definitions are principles. In 1957, Felix Biestek (an American priest and professor of social work) expounded seven principles of what he termed 'the casework relationship', based on what he saw as the needs of the people with whom social workers work:

- to be treated as an individual;
- to express feelings;
- to get sympathetic responses to problems;
- to be accepted as a person of worth;
- not to be judged;
- to make one's own choices and decisions;
- to have confidentiality respected.

Biestek summed up that the social worker 'is expected to be a firm footed realist and a clear eyed idealist'. Social work is a particularly paradoxical activity, sometimes described as 'contested' in that there is no general agreement about what it is. Biestek's principles illustrate this. They are sound principles, but they reflect just one facet of social work – the personal. A set of principles based on social work as broader than individual casework might read something like this:

- to feel empowered;
- to participate fully in the local community;
- to have differences respected and celebrated;
- to contribute to a just and equal society;
- not to be discriminated against;
- to achieve one's potential, not just individually but collectively;
- to have privacy.

Social work is an academic, scientific discipline as well as an activity. It is a young discipline and, as we shall see, has long depended on borrowings, in particular from sociology, psychology, social policy and social administration (its cognate disciplines). Philosophy, politics, economics and the law are influential, as are educational, ecological, anthropological and biological theories.

METAPHORS

Definitions are dry and wordy. A sideways view of social work can be gained through metaphor, which encourages us to make a comparison between two unlike things that, nevertheless, have something in common. For example, Biestek's notion that social workers are both firm-footed realists and clear-eyed idealists might suggest social workers as chameleons or contortionists.

Metaphors often rely on dark humour, as in 'rats leaving the sinking ship' to describe social workers taking redundancy at a time of budget cuts; or social work likened to a can of worms positioned behind a front door. Social work might be seen as a human satnav system, navigating people through their troubles towards their future. A common metaphor for social work in groups is that they are 'all in the same boat'.

Suggestions on an online site for objects to represent social work included a suit of armour, a mountain of paperwork, a blinking computer screen, a brick wall (for head-banging), a ball of tangled wool, becoming untangled if you are an optimist, and a two-headed coin, Mother Teresa on one side, Hitler the other (www. communitycare.co.uk/can-worms).

The English language has a fascination with collective nouns. There is a den of thieves and a worship of writers but no collective noun for social workers. A *lateness* of social workers would gently mock the well-known tendency for social workers to have a problem with the clock; or an *intention* of social workers to celebrate the gap that too often opens between hopeful purpose and hard reality.

THE SOCIAL WORK STORY

Storytelling is fundamental to human society and gives rise to the notion of *narrative* to describe the way we make sense of our personal and social histories. We develop narratives to give meaning to our histories, a thread that holds events together that might otherwise seem random and pointless. Sometimes these narratives go further than explanations and become the driving force; for example, a person has constructed a strong life script as someone who will marry young and have children, so they feel themselves to be a failure when they reach thirty-five without this happening.

Professions and organisations have narratives, too, though they are usually contested, in the sense that different groups hold to different stories. For instance, one narrative of the British National Health Service tells the story of a carefree, cheap and cheerful NHS beaten into its bowed and burdened current self. A competing narrative sees the NHS as arthritic and sclerotic, with a cure only possible with deep cuts and extensive free-market surgery to introduce competition. The one metaphor might be the NHS as a listed building, creaky, leaky and expensive to maintain, but nonetheless beautiful; for the other, it needs razing to the ground or at least the addition of a sumptuous privately funded wing (with acknowledgements to Sheldon and Macdonald, 2009: 16 for these two images).

How, then, might the social work story be cast? Let us take the four basic dramatic types to develop four plot lines for *Social Work: The Movie*. (Just to note that readers new to social work might like to return to these narratives later when you have more backstory.)

The first, *comedy-melodrama*, sees a triumph over adversity.

Plucky little Social Work, new on the scene and forever the Cinderella, actually survives against all the odds, gets written into key legislation and acquires recognition as a graduate profession. Although dominated by bigger brothers and sisters, Social Work quietly infiltrates their heads with social work ideas and values – so quietly that they don't even realise it.

The second narrative type is the *romantic saga*, in which there are recurring triumphs and setbacks.

So, the story starts with Lady Bountiful's transformative love affair with Freud and the psychoanalysts – or was it just a case of learned helplessness? The affair ends in the inevitable tears. On the rebound, Social Work renounces the Lady Bountiful title and finds brief happiness with Marx and the radicals and realises that the earlier relationship was a case of false consciousness; but pretty soon Social Work is caught two-timing with the Behaviourists. There are flirtations with Systems theory and other dalliances that bring only short-lived pleasures. It seems that Social Work falls at the feet of each passing fashion – structural, post-modern, solution-focused – until, weary and friendless, Social Work loses all allure and is forced to succumb to the prescriptions of Doctor Health. The audience is left with the hope that this is just the latest setback and that Social Work will rejuvenate and find a true self ...

Then there is *tragedy*, the fall into adversity.

Social Work stands face set square, like a Soviet statue, braving the hostile Forces of Reaction led by The Establishment. The battle for a unified social work profession is fought and Social Work emerges triumphant, with the biggest, fastest-growing budget on the block. But then things start to turn nasty. The battle for neighbourhood and locality-based work is lost. Social Work is accused of a series of child murders and the media whips up a vicious witch hunt. Social Work suffers a diaspora and is absorbed by warring tribes – the children and families, the adult services and the mental healths. Can Social Work regroup and find a way home ...

Finally, there is *irony-satire*, in which the outcomes are unexpected.

Social Work starts our story as a happy-go-lucky, easy-going free spirit, given to odd bursts of passion about following your instincts, doing your best by people and sticking to your principles. Social Work is an outdoors type. Gradually, by twist and turn through the story, Social Work somehow ends up in a dark office stuck behind a huge bank of computer screens. You should have seen it coming but somehow you didn't. Social Work is still remarkably chirpy, seems almost to have forgotten those passionate early speeches, rationalises the state of affairs.

Then, just as it seems all is going to end quietly but rather sadly, Tristan – hitherto, a minor character at the Ministry of Dark Forces – mistakenly has a bright idea: it would be ever such a good thing for Social Work to get out a bit. Everyone else at the Ministry has taken voluntary redundancy, so Tristan just goes ahead and signs an Instruction there and then. By no particular design or purpose, Social Work finds the doors opening and the wind blowing all the papers away and the light streaming in, blindingly. Social Work stands up, falteringly, and the audience feels a collective lump in its throat: can Social Work take those steps back into the light after all ...

These narratives tell the stories of social work primarily from a British perspective and in the Hollywood style; Bollywood treatments of Indian social work would read differently, but there would still be stories to tell.

ORIGINS OF SOCIAL WORK

A profession's history is important. It tells us, in part, why it looks as it presently does and it provides a yardstick to measure the ways in which the profession has changed. Knowledge of how it responded to challenges in the past can help to find better solutions in the present.

The teaching of the history of social work is on the decline, squeezed out of the curriculum by competing topics such as the Common Assessment Framework (to take an example from the UK). How much do social workers know of Helena Radinska's role in developing the first Polish social work school at an institute of higher learning in 1925 and her clandestine activities during the Second World War to help preserve social work values? And of Alice Salomon's pre-eminent role in the development of social work education and its international connections, and her decision to close her innovative Women's Academy in Berlin rather than obey Nazi demands to oust Jewish staff and students? Would they be surprised that Jane Addams, an early radical social worker in Chicago, was reported in the press of the time as the most dangerous woman in the United States? Clement Attlee, quoted earlier, has lost his identity as a social worker, overshadowed by later fame as the Labour Prime Minister at the creation of the British welfare state. The founding father of the Indian constitution, Dr Ambedkar, one of India's Untouchables, is known to Indians as a social worker, as are many of India's independence fighters. The loss of social work history from the curriculum risks impoverishing the profession.

As well as the people who tie social work to its history, we might wish to consider what historical sites would be 'listed' on a map of social work. Each country would have its own sites and artefacts. In the US, Jane Addams' Hull House in Chicago is, indeed, a museum to social work and a celebration of her work and that of her partner, Ellen Gates Starr. Toynbee Hall in London remains a living memorial to its reforming past and present. The radical roots of British history tend largely to be neglected and, similarly, it is unlikely that any social work heritage sites have a blue plaque.

EARLY REFORMIST ROOTS

Modern social work's foundations were solidly connected to poverty and destitution in the nineteenth century. Social work has consistently concerned itself with how to help people in these circumstances but it has long had different responses: whether to focus on the person in poverty or on the cause of the poverty or, indeed, on enlightening the wider world to the existence of the poverty, turning private troubles into public stories. These paths are not mutually exclusive, but they have tended to set the profession's hares running in different directions.

The Poor Law governed social attitudes to poverty in England over many centuries. The first Elizabethan Poor Law provided relief for each community's poor alongside other measures such as prevention of evictions, control of food supplies and prices, and securing labour practices. There was much poverty but little destitution. The agricultural and industrial revolutions saw the dismantling of these controls and a hardening of public attitudes towards poor people. By the nineteenth century, social obligations to the poor were vestigial, destitution was rife and seen as proof of idleness and moral failings.

The Victorian Poor Law established workhouses whose conditions were appalling, though with significant local variations, supposedly to make work more attractive than charity. Reformist elements concerned themselves with how best to administer the Poor Laws humanely and efficiently rather than to question them. Reformists were less concerned with poverty itself than in emphasising the mutual obligations between rich and poor in order to mitigate the worst effects. In short, the response to all this need was still rooted in a notion of individual charity.

Amongst the reforming pioneers were Octavia Hill, the Charity Organisation Society (COS) founded in 1869 and ancestor of the organisation now known as Family Action, the Barnetts at Toynbee Hall Settlement (founded 1884) and Dr Barnado, all based in London. The National Society for the Prevention of Cruelty to Children (NSPCC) was established at this time (1884). Jane Addams visited the Toynbee Hall settlement in the 1880s and, impressed by the work she saw as well as similar places in Germany, established Hull House settlement in Chicago in 1889.

These early reformers practised personalised approaches and they documented their work systematically, developing what we would now recognise as 'practice wisdom'. The significant role that systematic documentation has for the development of usable knowledge is an important lesson and one not always remembered.

We think of these early days as the beginnings of casework, a service tailored to individuals and their families and popularised by the work of Mary Richmond. However, what later became known as community work is also rooted in these times. 'The welfare and organisation of the district' was important both to the COS and to Toynbee Hall. Octavia Hill encouraged her workers (friendly visitors, as they were known) to live amongst the poor. Setting up workshops, bulk-buying schemes for tenants and campaigning for open spaces were all integral to the work of the pioneers, alongside individual and family casework. It is an enormous loss that these early beginnings, in which casework, family work, groupwork and community work were so well integrated, have not survived.

Working alongside other professions has a long history, too. The early social workers – almoners, probation workers and psychiatric social workers – were employed in settings where social work was secondary and they had to discover, as social workers do now, how best to make their specific social work contribution in places where social work is not well understood.

EARLY RADICAL ROOTS

These charity pioneers are now seen as essentially reformist rather than radical. For example, the COS opposed state provision as undermining what it saw as the Poor Law 'incentive' to self-improvement. However, they did hold firm beliefs about the *equality* of people (usually in the eyes of their God) and the rights as well as the obligations of individuals. They emphasised the need to treat people as equals, to develop friendships and even the power of love.

The enormous gap between the philanthropists and the poor with whom they worked can lead us to dismiss these sentiments as paternalistic and naive. However, we should see them in the context of their own time and understand how starkly different they were from prevailing attitudes, where poor people were condemned not just to poverty but for their supposed fecklessness. Compassion was, in its own way, quite radical. Toynbee Hall's current description of itself as having 'one foot in the establishment and the other amongst the poor' illustrates social work's position then as well as now.

The early reformers saw the existing system as essentially just and right but in need of some adjustment. Radicals saw the need for entirely different social and economic arrangements. The direct experience of the degradation of life in the slums led organised labour and social reformers like Beatrice and Sidney Webb to radical conclusions. No matter how great the individual help, they saw no way out for most of the urban poor, and they advocated changes in the law, for social protection and for collective action to strengthen labour. These were the beginnings of organised attempts to improve social conditions on a large scale.

The radical analysis – that poverty was structural and required fundamental measures and social change to be eradicated – was boosted by the early stirrings of social science knowledge. Until then there had been no knowledge from social science to challenge the ideology that supported the Poor Laws. *Life and Labour of the People of London,* one of the earliest such enquiries, was conducted by Charles Booth in 1883 and it found that one in three of the population lived in abject poverty with only the barest necessities, a much higher proportion than had been supposed. It was an early example of the power of social science to shock popular thinking and challenge generally accepted beliefs.

The clash between the charitable philanthropists and the social radicals is the continuing dilemma for social work in a nutshell. It is clear that there are some ills for which personalised action is not appropriate; and yet people who are the victims of these broader, social injustices want and need personalised help and cannot be abandoned.

SOCIAL WORK VALUES AND ETHICS

Values refer to the ideas and beliefs that we hold in value. Much of the time they are implicit, so their influence is not always evident. Conversely, values might be held explicitly yet not necessarily adhered to in practice. It is possible to believe one thing, say another and do a third.

Professional values are those values that are understood to be held in common by individual members of that profession. They are often systematised into codes of ethics or mission statements. Codes of practice are typically a mix of general principles to guide practice and prescriptions that aim to specify what a social worker ought to do. Weblinks to ethical codes are available at the end of this chapter.

Social work places emphasis on its values. Typically, the curriculum for a degree in social work will include a whole sequence of teaching on values and the assessment of the students' practice includes their values as well as their knowledge and skills. There is a large literature concerning social work values. Social workers regularly face situations of moral ambiguity, when 'the right thing' is often not self-evident and is seen to be dependent on the context. Values are also important because of the social control functions of social work. This places a duty on social work to clarify the ethical implications of its role and therefore how acceptable the exercise of social control is. Values regulate the power that comes from the social control aspects of social work.

Part of social work's narrative, as discussed earlier, is a strong belief that there are social work values held in common by the whole profession, a view seldom contested. However, a survey presenting social workers with a set of scenarios illustrating a possible dilemma elicited a wide variety of responses, both about how serious each situation was and what, if anything, should be done. How useful are these values if there are such wide differences in what social workers actually do, or is it possible to do different things whilst holding the same core values? Here are six of the situations:

1 A social worker becomes engaged to a person who until two months ago was a service user (client) of the agency that employs the social worker.
2 A social worker overclaims mileage allowance in order to fund a group for service users.
3 A social worker refuses to work with a same-sex couple because it contravenes their religious beliefs.
4 A social worker invites a service user to pray.
5 A social worker appears on local television with service users to publicise their plight.
6 A social worker is working as a dancer in a lap dancing club in their own time.

What are the assumed values of social work? The International Federation of Social Workers' statement in 2000 declared:

> Social work grew out of humanitarian and democratic ideals, and its values are based on respect for the equality, worth, and dignity of all people. Since its beginnings over a century ago, social work practice has focused on meeting human needs and developing human potential. Human rights and social justice serve as the motivation and justification for social work action. In solidarity with those who are disadvantaged, the profession strives to alleviate poverty and to liberate vulnerable and oppressed people in order to promote social inclusion. Social work values are embodied in the profession's national and international codes of ethics.

Are there any internal inconsistencies in these values? How do we incorporate differences when one value might conflict with another? As I write, there is debate about the stance that social workers in Uganda should take in relation to their government's criminalisation of homosexuality. We cannot reconcile the values that condemn same-sex relations with the values that underpin the rights of consenting adults. Social work values differences – but only those differences that it likes? In this, social work shares the classic liberal dilemma: is it right or possible to extend toleration to those who would rob you of the capacity to tolerate?

There is room to doubt, therefore, that the profession's values are the bedrock they are assumed to be and it is likely that social, political and religious subgroups have a greater influence on an individual than professional affiliation. Nor are social work values timeless. In Octavia Hill's time, drunkenness was seen as a failure of moral character, and by the 1960s as a lack of ego strength, and now it is more likely to be seen as the result of the social acceptability of binge drinking underpinned by the availability of cheap liquor. In my own span as a social worker I have witnessed a time when social work team members would go for a weekly lunch together at the pub, consume two pints of beer and several cigarettes, and drive off to visit clients in the afternoon; and a time, currently, when such behaviour would contravene the professional code of ethics and lead to termination of employment. The moral context for drunkenness (and other social problems) and the values that inform the social work response will continue to evolve and future generations will no doubt see their own values as immutable and timeless.

**

The following four sections briefly present the beginnings and evolution of social work knowledge, methods of practice, education and organisation. These topics are developed in greater detail in Chapters 4 and 5.

BEGINNINGS OF SOCIAL WORK KNOWLEDGE

The early pioneers developed knowledge for practice and this has continued to be the most productive mine for social work. Other kinds of knowledge – theory and model building – have been more fraught and too often appeared as a patchwork from other bodies of knowledge, such as sociology and psychology. If the scope of social work is as broad as the human and social condition we can see why it has proved difficult to agree a common basis of knowledge.

USABLE KNOWLEDGE

In nineteenth-century England, Octavia Hill and the women visitors who worked under her guidance documented their work. What would otherwise have been fleeting experiences became the rudiments of practice, events turned into usable knowledge. These enduring records helped social work to become established as a recognisable, discrete activity.

At a time of great advance in machinery – the steam engine, the motorcar and the beginnings of mechanical flight – it is not surprising that there was optimism for discoveries to be made about the mechanisms of society. Social conditions were mapped by scientific investigation. However, it was the mechanisms of the mind that came to dominate much of the middle twentieth century.

Mary Richmond's *Social Diagnosis* (1917) was one breakthrough in conceptualising social work, though its significance has been exaggerated compared to continental European social work pioneers such as Alice Salomon. Again, we see the significance of social work records in helping to theorise practice for transmission from one generation of social worker to another. American social work was subsequently heavily influenced by psychodynamic theory, in which an individual is understood by their psychological history and their unconscious motivations. These theories proved attractive, since they gave the individual practitioner an active role and the seeming possibility of bringing about change. What had been a moral failing in the times of the Poor Law was now a character disorder, with the same individualistic and moralistic undertones.

Private and voluntary social work agencies were the norm in the US and, in the competition for funds, there was a need to demonstrate effectiveness. Out of this developed the American tradition of large-scale controlled trials such as Cabot's delinquency prevention study in the 1930s. This set the pattern for ambitious experimental programmes that produced disappointing results for social work. Increases in knowledge exposed the level of uncertainty rather than providing the profession with comfortable answers and *usable* knowledge. There were some notable exceptions such as Bowlby, whose studies demonstrated the infant's need for consistent maternal care and theorised the processes of attachment and bonding. The findings were published at a time when Children's Departments were establishing themselves in early 1950s Britain, so Bowlby's work was well-timed and highly applicable.

In addition to attachment, key concepts in the post-war social work years were separation, loss, deprivation, trauma, alienation, inadequacy and delinquency. Social workers' clients were seen as damaged people in one respect or another, and these key notions all point to a 'weaknesses' model, though it was never termed this, that focused on what is wrong and not functioning. This contrasts with the later development of a strengths perspective. The strengths model has the premise that many of the people who are seen as struggling are, given their extraordinary circumstances, surviving remarkably well. A parent caring on her own for four children, each of whom has many health and social problems, living in a cramped flat with a minimal income might be coping rather better than her social worker would in those circumstances.

SERVICE USER KNOWLEDGE

Knowledge derived from the direct experience of working with service users or clients has long been central to social work, but a significant development has been the emphasis placed on their expertise and what is sometimes described as their 'lived experience'. Service users have become more their own authors, not just in recounting their own stories but as definers of social work knowledge and as members of formal social work research teams. The derivation of social work knowledge is, therefore, understood to be diverse – from the experiences of service users and social workers, and from formal and informal research.

ROOTS OF MODELS AND METHODS

SOCIAL AND MEDICAL MODELS

When drunkenness is called a social disease, as it was by the Barnetts of Toynbee Hall, a medical model is being used to explain a social phenomenon. The medical model uses the scientific method of history-taking, examination, diagnosis, treatment and prognosis. It is an individualised model designed for interventions that are physical. By contrast, the social model focuses on social context and the social meaning of what are seen as phenomena not diseases.

The roots of these two models can be seen in the differences between the individualism of the reformers and the social solutions of the radicals. The dominance of psychodynamic thinking saw the ascendancy of the medical model in social work until the radical social work movement of the 1970s and the disability movement of the 1980s reinstated the social model in social work practice.

Let us consider the phenomenon of childhood obesity to illustrate how the two models work. In the medical model the individual child receives a variety of possible treatments following diagnosis: surgery, counselling, diet education, medication, etc. The social model sees child obesity as the manifestation of broader social phenomena such as food industry policies (sugars added to processed foods, large portion sizes to justify higher pricing and advertising techniques), transport policies (cheap car travel adds traffic to the streets and walking is perceived as dangerous), food pricing (junk food is cheap compared to fresh fruit), school budgets (schools install fizzy drink machines to supplement cuts to their budgets), etc.

The two models are not mutually exclusive – the one focuses on reducing symptoms and the other attempts to eradicate the causes – but methods of practice are more easily constructed around the medical model than they are around the social model, the latter requiring political action, often at a global level. This helps to explain the continuing strength of the medical model.

EVOLUTION OF SOCIAL WORK EDUCATION

Many of the social work pioneers realised the need to train their volunteers and workers. The model was apprenticeship until Miss Sewell, warden of the Women's University Settlement, started lectures in 1895. These focused on what to do in practice, and they gradually grew into other areas. Even so, many staff remained untrained. The Charity Organisation Society started a school of sociology in London in 1903 with a two-year course, amalgamating with the London School of Economics in 1912. The course included periods of practical work in agencies. Social work courses were started at Birmingham and Liverpool universities in the early 1900s. The costs involved meant that these courses largely recruited middle-class young women. In 1936 the first publicly financed training scheme in Britain, the Probation Training Board, was established.

A formal social work training programme with an emphasis on practical work rather than academic subjects was established by the New York Charities Organisation Society in partnership with Columbia University in 1898, with the Chicago Settlement developing educational programmes from 1901. The first Irish social worker trained under Octavia Hill in 1899 and the first Irish diploma course was at Trinity College, Dublin, in 1934 and a four-year honours degree in 1962.

The University of Birmingham announced the following series of lectures for the year 1908–9, including arrangements for field visits. The fee for the whole course was £6.6s.0d (£6.30p or about $10) which included membership of the university library.

THE BRITISH CONSTITUTION – Professor Masterman
Twenty lectures Fee £1.1s.0d [£1.05p]
ENGLISH LOCAL GOVERNMENT – Professor Masterman
Twenty lectures Fee £1.1s.0d [£1.05p]
INDUSTRIAL HISTORY – Professor Ashley
Ten lectures Fee 10s.6d [52½p]
ECONOMIC ANALYSIS – Professor Ashley
Seventeen lectures Fee £1.1s.0d [£1.05p]
METHOD OF STATISTICS – Professor Ashley
Twenty lectures Fee £1.1s.0d [£1.05p]
INDUSTRIAL CONDITIONS – George Shan
Twenty lectures Fee £1.1s.0d [£1.05p]
SANITATION AND HYGIENE – John Robertson
Twenty lectures Fee £1.1s.0d [£1.05p]
LAW FOR SOCIAL WORKERS – Frank Tillyard
Five lectures Fee 5/-[25p]
AIMS AND METHODS OF SOCIAL WORK – Professor Muirhead
Five lectures Fee 5/-[25p]

In connection with particular parts of the course arrangements will be made for visits under competent escort to the following institutions etc.:

ADMINISTRATION

(a) **POOR LAW** – Workhouse – Infirmary – Receiving House for Children – Cottage Homes – Epileptic Colony – Home for Defective Children
(b) **EDUCATION** – Infant and Elementary Schools – Schools for Defective, Blind, Deaf and Crippled Children – Technical and Art Schools

(c) **JUSTICE** – Children's Court – The Probation System – Reformatory and Industrial Schools

SANITATION AND HYGIENE

Housing improvements – Hospitals (General and Special) – Elementary Schools (Hygiene and Domestic Teaching)

INDUSTRIAL CONDITIONS

Factories – industries and domestic workshops

A certificate will be granted after examination on the completion of the curriculum. In order to encourage the attendance of suitable students of limited means, who might not otherwise be able to devote their whole time for a year to such a course of preparation, it is proposed to offer free tuition to a limited amount of students (no more than six). Applications for this remission should be accompanied by a confidential statement as to previous career, aim of study, and means.

With thanks to Ann Davis for permission to reproduce this syllabus from 'Celebrating 100 Years of Social Work at University of Birmingham', 2008

The first international organisation for social work education was established in 1928, to become the International Association of Schools of Social Work (IASSW), with Alice Salomon as the president.

In British social work we take for granted the distinctions between qualified social workers who must be registered to hold the title of social worker, and assistants, trainees, ancillary staff and volunteers. Currently, the distinction is often made between social work and social care staff. These distinctions only started to become clear in the 1960s as the shortage of social workers became evident and the numbers of training programmes increased.

DEVELOPMENT OF SOCIAL WORK ORGANISATION

In order to provide help as effectively as possible, the COS developed organisational structures, including offices covering local neighbourhoods. The multiplicity of charities made it necessary to find ways to co-ordinate activities; Attlee noted in 1920 that the list of societies working just with blind people covered twenty-four pages of the Annual Charities Register. Social workers began to be employed in the welfare departments of industries, such as the Jacobs biscuit factory in 1906. Social workers no longer have factory locations in the UK, but this remains a feature of social work in some countries. In the US, for instance, they are employed in Employee Assistance Programs (EAPs) in large corporations and businesses.

The impact of the Second World War and, in particular, the large-scale evacuation of children from urban centres (3 million children were removed to the countryside) was the spur for local government in the UK to begin employing social workers. By the end of the war seventy local authorities were doing just that. The Curtis Report (1946) revealed the chaotic organisation of the various services involved with children and arrived at conclusions about co-ordinated services that continue to be rediscovered, now referred to as 'joined up services'. The Children Act created children's departments in every local authority and the role of child care officer. For the first time, social workers were being employed in increasing numbers and the expansion was driven by the state.

The Seebohm Report (1968) was a defining moment for the organisation of social work. This amalgamated the children's, welfare and mental welfare services into single Social Services Departments (SSD) and, in Scotland, probation and after-care services too. Most SSDs organised themselves into neighbourhood teams and there was a flowering of community social work or 'patchwork'. For the next decade or two, the four methods of social work (see p. 12) were as nearly integrated as they had ever been since the early pioneers.

Although the construction of a welfare state resulted in growing numbers of social workers employed by the state (over 90 per cent at its height in the UK), in countries like the US where state funding was paltry, the organisation of social work continued in private and voluntary agencies. A two-tier system in the US consigned public services to the last resort for the uninsured.

PROFESSIONAL ORGANISATION

Social workers began to organise themselves into professional organisations. The seven organisations that consolidated themselves in 1955 into the National Association of Social Workers (US) and the seven that formed the British Association (BASW) in 1970 (right-hand column) give an insight into social work's professional roots:

American Association of Social
Workers (AASW)
American Association of Psychiatric
Social Workers (AAPSW)
American Association of Group
Workers (AAGW)
Association for the Study of
Community Organization (ASCO)
American Association of Medical
Social Workers (AAMSW)
National Association of School Social
Workers (NASSW)
Social Work Research Group
(SWRG)

Association of Child Care
Officers (ACCO)
Association of Family
Caseworkers
Association of Psychiatric
Social Workers
Association of Moral
Welfare Workers
Association of Social
Workers
Institute of Medical Social
Workers
Society of Mental Welfare
Officers

New professional organisations of social workers continue to be formed, such as the Georgian Association of Social Workers, established in 2004 and with a 2011 membership of 200. At an international level, the International Federation of Social Workers (IFSW) was established in 1956, a successor to the International Permanent Secretariat of Social Workers, which was founded in Paris in 1928 at the first international conference of social workers, which saw nearly 2,500 people attend from forty-two countries.

WELFARE

Welfare is a complex term. Sometimes it refers to a broad notion of general well-being. In the UK it is more likely to be taken for the range of social and health provision that comprises the welfare state; in continental Europe, social protection, social security or the social state; and in the US it is a narrow term referring to a financial safety net only for poor people who cannot manage otherwise. European notions of welfare are based on notions of social solidarity and the mutual responsibilities that people have towards one another in the community and the nation state as a whole. Despite frequent talk of the 'Anglo-Saxon model', the UK is far closer to continental Europe than to the US in this respect. Child death rates (from unintentional and intentional injury) are 0.24 per 100,000 in England and 3.67 in the US. Might the different welfare models explain this very large discrepancy? The political left sees welfare as an arm in the redistribution of resources; the radical right is opposed to welfare on the principle that it violates the absolute right of individuals to their property and wealth.

WELFARE STATE

The construction of the British welfare state by the Labour government in the years immediately following the Second World War was an exceptional achievement, especially given the austerity of the time. A National Health Service free at the point of delivery was established in the face of hostility from much of the medical profession and the opposition Conservative party. The Poor Law was at last replaced by National Assistance, with state pensions for all and a comprehensive scheme for unemployment benefit.

The state was firmly at the centre of provision and this provided the opportunity for large-scale employment of social workers to help make the welfare state a reality. We take this for granted, yet a belief that there would be no need for social workers could have prevailed. With a welfare state designed to eradicate want and hardship, what need for social work? This was the official view in the socialist utopia of the Soviet Union, that in a just social system (communism) social problems will disappear. However, *Social Work in Britain*, Eileen Younghusband's 1951 review, was influential in promoting social work, celebrating social workers' contribution in the war and noting their part in the new Children's Departments and in the health service.

WELFARE MODELS

Although the establishment of the British welfare state was a victory for the radical tradition at the level of policy, social work practice remained largely individualist and reformist. Social work has found it difficult to articulate its response to the various models of welfare that have developed in the post-war period: *command and control*, with its reliance on centralisation and hierarchy; *market*, with price, profit and competition as the driving forces; and *networks*, with an emphasis on trust, reciprocity and co-ordination. The first model was dominant until the 1980s, the second model has been ascendant since then, and the third is still largely on the drawing board.

SOCIAL WORK AND SOCIAL PROBLEMS

The notion of a social problem is modern. In mediæval times misery, poverty and sickness were personal calamities, not social problems. Growing urban populations and the parallel growth of knowledge fostered the notion that these were *social* problems, amenable to collective action and requiring social policies to eradicate them. Collective action became state action, with the creation of the welfare state providing security 'from cradle to grave'. The aim was nothing short of abolishing the 'five giants' of want, squalor, ignorance, unemployment and ill-health. It was these institutions of the welfare state that suckled the modern social work profession.

SOCIAL AND GLOBAL PROBLEMS

The five giants were tamed rather than eradicated by the welfare state and poverty was 'rediscovered' in the 1960s. Other problems were highlighted, notably racism and sectarianism, domestic violence and child abuse, migration, crime, drug and alcohol use, levels of mental illness, and the effects of institutionalisation. Some 'problems' were removed, at least in the eyes of the law, such as homosexuality.

Different sections of the community are likely to highlight alternative social issues as problematic: are 'family values' a social problem? Are out-of-town shopping malls a social problem? Smoking in public places? What is anti-social behaviour: youths gathering around a bus-stop playing loud music or large multinationals failing to pay their taxes?

In recent times there has been an increasing recognition of the significance of global problems. The five giants are far from abolished at a global level and, whereas the rise of fascism was a global concern for social workers in the 1930s, people trafficking is likely to top international social work concerns in the 2010s. The impact of the globalisation of the world economy and of climate change may seem well beyond the purview of social work, but the fallout is exactly what social work has to work with. We return to these themes in Chapter 6.

SOCIAL POLICY AND WICKED PROBLEMS

Social policy is the study of social welfare and its relationship to politics and society. It is concerned with social planning and administration, financing, and, in one sense, social work might be described as applied social policy – an application that is critical and reflective. In the limited space available, perhaps the best way to consider the intricacies of social work and social policy is by way of an example:

> Social workers are finding it very hard to recruit foster carers in one particular area. They wonder why the idea of foster care should be so unattractive to people in these neighbourhoods, as they are fairly affluent. They pep up their advertising and recruitment drives. In fact, the disappointing level of recruitment has nothing to do with foster care itself. The absence of affordable housing in this relatively affluent area means that there are fewer families with spare rooms who might in other ocircumstances like to offer foster placements. So, the problem is affordable housing, or rather a lack of it, not an absence of interest in fostering. The social policies that have led to a lack of affordable housing have now become a problem for social work.

This is an example of a 'wicked problem'. This term is used to indicate the complexity of social problems; that information is incomplete, perhaps even contradictory, and it is changing all the time. Work to alleviate one problem might create others. Seen in this light, the steady-state idea of careful social planning is flawed. In the presence of a wicked problem there is a temptation to throw up our arms in despair, but there are always 'best available solutions', even for superwicked problems like climate change. The social work team in the foster care example above can at least begin to refine their strategies in the light of their new knowledge.

We will see in the next chapter how social policy is often shaped by individual high-profile cases rather than by a careful arrangement of the facts.

SOCIAL JUSTICE AND SOCIAL INCLUSION

Social justice is an underlying principle of much social work. It is distributive, in the sense that it concerns the proportions of give and take in society, the fair shares. It is represented in the maxim popularised by Marx, 'from each according to his ability, to each according to his need'.

As well as the injustices in social and economic arrangements, many social workers are motivated by the injustice that arises from different life chances and opportunities, whether these are social, psychological or biological. The hard bit is working out what this means in practice and social workers are frequently in the frontline of these kinds of decision, charged with understanding what is or would be just. In the field of juvenile offending they might be directly involved in a particular type of justice known as restorative, bringing those harmed and those responsible for the harm together, with a view to helping everyone affected to play a part in repairing the harm.

The idea of social justice starts from a position of equality, that everyone has the right to a fair share. Most Western democracies subscribe to an idea of equal rights and equal opportunities, though they vary in the degree to which they adopt policies to achieve this. The reformist wing of social work subscribes to equal opportunity, but the radical and social democratic wing goes further towards redistributive justice, for example using progressive taxation to reallocate wealth in society.

More recently social justice has been reframed as social inclusion and there is concern that the emphasis has changed from the need to change social structures to a focus on including people with the help of various social programmes. Social work, with one foot in the mainstream and the other in the marginalised world, has a particular duty to work with socially excluded groups and to bring the two worlds of included and excluded together.

Care has to be taken not to define 'hard to reach' groups solely in mainstream terms. For example, deaf people might be seen as socially excluded, whilst they actually have a very inclusive community of their own; it is just that it is separate from the mainstream hearing community.

CARE AND CONTROL

When I ask would-be social work students why they want to become social workers they frequently relate this to a generalised desire to help and a sense of caring. I have yet to meet somebody who has said that they want to exercise social control. It can be disconcerting when they become aware of the powers given to social workers and expectations that they will exercise them.

The balance between care and control is a fine one and it changes over time. The balance expected of social workers reflects the broader social balance between care and control. As Western societies have become economically more liberal they have become correspondingly more socially authoritarian. Technological advances have aided the growth of 'the surveillance society' and given tools for micro-management, a feature of the new authoritarianism. An example of the impact on social work is the emphasis on child protection at the expense of prevention work.

One response to the new social authoritarianism has been a reassertion of *relationship-based* social work. As the name suggests, this is an attempt to restore the balance away from coercive social work to a practice based on co-operation, with a working alliance between workers and service users. This is similar to the notion of *self-determination*.

POWER AND OPPRESSION

A seminal study in the early 1970s, *The Client Speaks*, exposed the disparity between the social workers' perceptions of what they were doing and the clients' views. The former thought they were working on the clients' family and personal relationships and the latter that they were receiving financial help, albeit with some preliminary talking. In fact, this was a failure on the part of the social workers to understand the impact of their power, as clients were playing the therapy game as part of what they saw as an unspoken compact which resulted in the desired financial rewards.

The radical social work tradition found expression from the 1980s in an analysis of power relations in society, especially in relation to gender and race/ethnicity. Anti-racist, anti-discriminatory and anti-oppressive practices focus on the personal, cultural and structural discrimination experienced by social minorities such as women, black people, old people, the gay community, disabled people and some religious groups. Children and poor people were seldom identified as oppressed minorities and 'the discourse' moved away from a class-based analysis. The term 'minoritised' is sometimes used in recognition that minorities like women can be numerically superior.

Prejudice at a personal level had long been understood, but the framework of power and oppression helped to understand systemic oppression. The challenge for social work, as ever, is how to use this knowledge in everyday practice.

> Let us take the example of an eleven-year-old black boy excluded from his school because he wore his hair in braided cornrows. The school only allowed 'short back and sides' and claimed other styles encourage gang culture. What should the school social worker do? Focus on working with the school to help it understand that cornrows are the 'short back and sides' for many Afro-Caribbean families, and aim to change the school's policy? Or work with the boy and his family to persuade them to change his hair style so that his schooling does not suffer any more? The reformist tradition in social work would tend to the latter and the radical tradition to the former. Neither excludes the other, of course.

CRITICAL SOCIAL POLICY: THE EXAMPLE OF BENEFIT FRAUD

The modern benefits system is not dissimilar to the Poor Law in that it is intended to provide relief to those who, in Tawney's words, have 'fallen by the wayside'. Hostility to the benefits system chimes remarkably closely with complaints about relief under the Poor Law: that it encourages idleness, that it forces up wage rates and that accepting it is proof of moral inferiority.

Tackling benefit fraud became a high-profile mission for the UK Coalition government in 2010, proclaiming 'zero tolerance', sometimes referred to as the criminalisation of poverty. Amidst severe cuts, it involved the recruitment of 200 extra anti-fraud officers and an additional £425m funding over four years. Financial rewards were proposed for people who tipped off the fraud investigation service; these could be anonymous and without consequence to the person providing the information, even if found to be malevolent. The UK national benefit fraud hotline receives 600 calls a day, in addition to the online report-a-benefit-thief service. (Much of the statistical information on benefits fraud comes from *The Guardian* (G2, 1/2/11, pp. 6–11).)

This campaign was launched at a time when benefit fraud was at a historical low – just 0.6 per cent of all claimants. Even this figure was inflated, as the government fraudulently included those whose claims were made as a result of a genuine error, often by the official managing the claim, as the system is exceptionally complex.

One might expect those who investigate fraud to be the most condemnatory, but contact with the individual people involved leads them to an understanding of *why* the fraud is committed: extreme poverty, debt, a drug or alcohol dependency, Christmas presents for the kids, etc. It is exactly this kind of personal contact that has a strong influence on social workers. It is easier to condemn a group of people from a safe distance, but social workers get close to the people and the situations they work with, in contrast to a political plutocracy that is distant from the people whom they condemn.

UNINTENDED CONSEQUENCES

Social policies frequently have consequences that were unintended. The Speenhamland system of poor relief in the eighteenth century was designed to provide work for agricultural labourers during times of want; but the organisation of the funding resulted in it becoming a subsidy by local town trades for agricultural labour and therefore very unpopular. From this was born the workhouse.

In current times, the policy of *personalisation* in the UK was supposed to bypass cumbersome processes and make things simpler and more direct (see Chapter 3 for more details). However, a poll of social workers in 2010 revealed a majority for whom personalisation had increased bureaucracy, as well as the unanticipated costs of redundancy payments when personal assistants' employment was terminated.

Unintended consequences are particularly bleak in the relationship between crime and drug policies. Urine drug tests introduced into prisons in the 1990s led to a shift from cannabis use to heroin because heroin cleared the system more quickly than cannabis. Out on the streets, the criminalisation of drug use, rather than its legal regulation, drives up the price so that an estimated 90 per cent of crime is associated with the need to pay this artificially high price. Social workers pick up the pieces of these mistaken social policies.

AGENTS OF THE STATE?

A lively debate in the social work trade press concerned the role of social pedagogues (see page 39) in helping the state intrude into the family – at a time when the state in question was Nazi. Whatever the truth in this proposition, the idea that social work polices the underclass is not new.

Can social work exacerbate social problems? We have until now seen the reformist elements in social work as, at worst, benign and well-motivated in their desire to alleviate suffering. However, even in 1920, Attlee was noting that the distribution of doles (money, blankets, soup, etc.) had its effect on the local wages, making workers less ready to stand out for higher wages and employers less prepared to pay them. Local rents rose because of crowding, so landlords were in effect subsidised by the local charities. Whilst it is unlikely that the ministrations of social workers in the post-war period have prevented the Revolution, the pressure cooker metaphor for British society is often used to explain the Establishment's talent for survival. Reforms are just sufficient to prevent insurrection but not enough to make any real difference; and, in the pressure cooker imagery, social work is part of the release valve.

Social workers need an understanding of the relevance of social policy to their practice, and also the role their own practice plays in the solution or, indeed, as part of the problem.

IDEOLOGY

Social workers by and large see themselves as pragmatists and, certainly, successful work in a large bureaucracy requires compromise and negotiation. However, if ideology is about conformity to a set of beliefs that offer a comprehensive vision, social work has been, and continues to be, influenced by some quite different ideologies. The principal ones are reviewed briefly.

RELIGION

Organised religion has often been at the heart of the moral order, defining the social obligations of a community, and so it remains in some societies. Charity is common to all of the world's major religions and religious motivation was strong amongst the early social work reformers. Religion and social work both concern themselves with the position of the individual in society and grapple with moral ambiguities. In many Western countries, such as the UK, the charity relationship between giver and receiver became suspect and the creation of a welfare state removed these obligations and gave them to the state, where they became embedded as human rights rather than religious duties.

Social work has a role to play in working with people who suffer discrimination or persecution because of their religion; in particular, to counter the growing Islamophobia in Western countries. Social work itself is a largely secular rather than a spiritual activity in the UK, more likely to be humanist than religious. Although there are many socially liberal religions whose members have been at the forefront of social reform, fundamentalist religious activity is often associated with beliefs that are at odds with mainstream social work values. An example of this is the obsession of some religious factions with sexual rather than spiritual life and, in particular, the hostility to same-sex relationships. Perhaps it is helpful to draw a distinction between spirituality on the one hand and religious ideology on the other and to emphasise that the notion of faith is not tied exclusively to religious faith.

CAPITAL, LABOUR AND COMMODIFICATION

Few tricks of the unsophisticated intellect are more curious than the naive psychology of the business man, who ascribes his achievements to his unaided efforts, in blind unconsciousness of a social order without whose continuous support and vigilant protection he would be a lamb bleating in the desert.

R.H. Tawney, *Religion and the Rise of Capitalism*,
Harmondsworth: Pelican, 1926: 264

Economic relationships between individuals and the state spring from prevailing notions about the nature of social relations. At what point is it right that individual initiatives should be curtailed by social controls, and private interests subordinated to the public good?

Painstaking social and economic research should provide us with informed answers to these fundamental questions and to some extent it does. We know that there has never been a famine in a democracy, that societies with the greatest gaps between the wealthy and the poor are less economically productive and that their populations are generally less contented (not just the poorer classes). We know that 'trickledown economics' does not work – it was used to justify huge wealth accumulating in the hands of the very few by virtue of that wealth trickling down to benefit all social classes. It doesn't. We know that poverty causes misery and shortens lives but that there is a point at which greater wealth does not bring more contentment. We know these things yet they are largely ignored in policymaking. This is because ideology plays a much larger part than social and economic knowledge.

The balance between individual and society recalibrates with time and place. Arguments for greater social controls and regulation were considerably strengthened in Western democracies by the experiences of the world wars and the relationship of the citizen to the state changed radically. However, since the 1980s policy has gone into reverse so that, to use Milton Friedman's phrase, there is now 'socialism for the rich and free enterprise for the rest'. In recent years, corporate ideology has been dominant.

Prevailing economic and social relations have a significance for social work in many ways. The wealth of a nation determines the availability of resources to provide employment, education and good health for its population, as well as direct funding for social work. However, it is the distribution of these resources that determines whether they *are* used for these purposes. The rates of homicide and child mortality and the absence of health care for large numbers in the richest country in the world stand as stark testimony to the significance of the extent to which Gross Domestic Product is *distributed* (or not) rather than its overall size. As we might expect, the US public social work services are poorly resourced, residual and of low status; and access to the higher-status private practice social work is controlled by the US insurance business.

Continental Europe and the UK have stronger traditions of state welfare and solidarity models of social and economic relations, though this has been steadily weakening, especially in the UK. A process with the ugly name of commodification has taken a hold of social relations. Examples are everywhere: all over the walls of my local gym there are signs exhorting us to REFER A FRI£ND, the semiotics cleverly suggesting that our friends are also a source of income. When I return to my home city of Sheffield I am welcomed back to the city boundary courtesy of a local company, and the flower beds on the local roundabout are, so a sign informs us, maintained by another local business.

Whole cities and neighbourhoods that used to do their own welcoming and maintenance are now available for commercial exploitation, and so it is for social work. Social care is described as an industry, universities have core business and large tracts of public service are being treated as commodities ripe for profit. However, there are many parts of social work that are unattractive in economic terms, just as there are bus routes to nether regions that need subsidy from the popular ones. Will commodification inevitably lead to a two-tier service, with less attractive forms of social work following the US model of an impoverished residual service – the deserving and undeserving of the nineteenth century transformed into the profitable and unprofitable of the twenty-first?

If social work is itself a commodity, who might be said to 'own' it? The profession itself has been working hard to develop a radical model of partnership with the people who use social work and other people with a direct interest ('stakeholders' in business management talk). It is an important experiment, but in danger of being swept away if social work finds itself sold off, wholesale or in bits, to commercial interests. These interests are changing shape, too: the extent to which social enterprises will in the end revert to economic enterprises is yet to be seen. (see pages 120–1 for further discussion.)

In summary, if we have to single out one pre-eminent condition that favoured the rise of social work in Western societies it was organised labour. It is no coincidence that as organised labour has weakened since the 1980s, the breach between rich and poor has widened dramatically. The prospect of labour, in this case social work practitioners, truly owning social work remains elusive.

COMMUNITY

In the social work story, the ideology of community is generally positive. Communities provide support to their members and activists fight off the excesses of local and central powers. There is an alternative ideology that casts communities as reactionary, ready to exclude and ostracise those who do not conform to their rigid norms. Both narratives of community are possible, as well as many others. Social work recognises the significance of communities and the task of discovering how to help them achieve their potential.

As an 'apple pie' term, community's latest sibling in the UK is the Big Society. Everyone has a vague idea about what this could mean, but one cynic noted that it is the dismissing of people who work in libraries, citizens advice bureaux and schools so that they will have more free time to volunteer in libraries, citizens advice bureaux and schools. (Acknowledgements to Simon Hoggart, *The Guardian*, 10/2/11.)

Community has become associated less with geography and more with interest. Greater physical and virtual mobility has spawned communities of interest and of practice. These communities can be a resource for the people who use social work (for instance, internet support groups) and for social workers themselves, such as professional special interest groups, sometimes called communities of practice.

A FEW -ISMS

Freudianism and Marxism were the most influential -isms following the middle years of the twentieth century, but feminism has had the single most significant impact on social work. The role of the women's suffrage movement was critical, like organised labour, to the early development of social work. The focus on electoral inclusion is well known, but the suffragette movement also forced the political establishment to consider issues of family welfare and women in employment, a precursor of the later feminist slogan 'the personal is political'. These were significant issues for social work, both for its practice and for its practitioners, very largely female.

Social work remains a highly female profession, not just in the raw numbers of women employed but in the quality and nature of social work as a profession and a practice. Given this, and social work's critical social policy orientation, it is not surprising that social work has been highly influenced by feminist theories and approaches. The emphasis on equality, fairness at home and work, and a critique of patriarchal societies all chime with social work values. Feminism's emphasis on relationships, especially in terms of power relations, and empowerment through partnerships amongst equals, makes it a significant paradigm for social work research.

One lacuna in social work practice is the missing male, in the workforce (though it will come as no surprise that men become more prevalent in social work management and senior academic posts), and more particularly in the clientele. The evidence suggests that by far the most typical social work encounter is female to female and that the vast majority of men have no contact with social work. We will return to gender and social work on pages 85–6.

Social work has had an ambiguous relationship with *post-modernism*. The interplay between the personal and the political and the notion that knowledge is not linear but constructed, deconstructed and reconstructed chimes with social work: everything is fluid and contestable, nothing is certain and identities are continually re-forming. However, there are tensions. Social work is a creature of modernism, that is, the optimistic belief in big, radical solutions that was epitomised by the welfare state and which, let us not forget, was enormously successful. Post-modernist thinking dissolves the idea of collective solidarity that has been so central to social work and it lends intellectual authority to the fractured individualism that is corrosive of social work.

MANAGERIALISM

Whether social work was to be primarily reformist or radical, no-one expected it to become a bystander. In the past two decades in the UK and US, a third tide in social work affairs has overwhelmed the reform and radical swells: case management. The social worker as case manager saw the gradual retreat of much social work practice from direct contact with clients to managing a package of care.

The introduction of management practices from the private sector into the public sector in the UK began during the Thatcher years (1980s) and has gathered rather than lost momentum. This policy saw managers rather than practitioners becoming the main instrument of social policy. Previously, social work was based on the relationship between the social worker and the client and the success of the work was internally driven: that is, successful work was defined by the worker and client together. However, it became externally driven, with success measured by targets set by the employing agency, which, in turn, reacted to government policies. Even the permissions to start and continue the work became externally driven by 'eligibility criteria' that were determined outside the individual social worker's professional responsibility. This system of micro-management, combined with the practices imported from the profit-driven private sector, is referred to as managerialism.

The managerialist approach prioritises procedures and targets over professional values and standards and it stresses compliance and rule-governed behaviour rather than critical analysis and reflection. Private sector management must capture data about production in order to secure a profit for the shareholders; a similar management strategy in the public sector has tended to value those things that are easy to count, with resources 'objectively' allocated on the basis of these counts. Managerialist practice therefore values quantitative measures over qualitative ones. An illustration of this is the value placed on an assessment completed within a prescribed time period rather than the quality of the assessment, still less a questioning of the assessment system itself.

Despite biting critiques of its inappropriate application to the public services and much hand-wringing at the effect on professional confidence and the gridlock levels of bureaucracy, managerialism continues to dominate. It offers an illusion of control which, unfortunately, diverts from the real task of managing uncertainty.

REORGANISING SERVICES

A feature of managerialism is the regular reorganisation of social work services. These restructurings are sometimes in response to changes driven by central government and at other times the whim of an incoming director wanting to make a mark. The absence of democracy in the workplace means that executive teams in most agencies wield near-feudal power and consultations need only be tokenistic. Perhaps observers a hundred years hence will reflect on the current times with the same astonishment we show at the disenfranchisement of women a century ago.

The costs of reorganisation in terms of lost productivity, to use the language of business, are rarely reckoned, though an Organisation for Economic Co-operation and Development (OECD) Report in 2011 estimated that each 'reform' of the UK National Health Service costs two years of improvements in quality. Despite the NHS being classed by the OECD as world-beating, reorganisations continue. The lack of an evidence base for the effectiveness of reorganisation suggests that it is an ideological pursuit. Indeed, Maoism is the nearest ideological reference point (though most Chief Executives would be astonished to read this), as the regular breaking up of teams and reassignment under new managers is a perfect policy to unsettle and destabilise a profession and to rattle its self-confidence.

Reorganisations turn the energies of an agency inwards. The self-obsession generated by the processes of reorganising are an irrelevance to service users, whose lives do not conform to organisational structures, past, present or planned.

THE COUSINS

In carving an identity for itself, social work has had to position itself amongst the family of professions. Some of social work's nearest relatives in the early days now seem quite remote: for example, Octavia Hill's model integrated social work and housing work in ways that have never been bettered, but housing work has lost much of its social concerns to become a technical competence.

Social work expanded to encompass probation work, residential work, community work and education welfare and the lists of professional associations that merged to form integrated social work associations (see earlier) indicate the wide range of cousins brought into the fold. Social work 'lost' housing management, personnel management and youth employment some while ago, and then in more recent times probation work, residential work and community work slipped away in England. The profession is in danger of disaggregating into its specialisms and we shall explore the growing power of health and education over social work in Chapter 6.

SOCIAL PEDAGOGY

Social work has a continental European cousin called social pedagogy. The work of social pedagogues focuses on the broad education and care of children and they often work with the same groups of children on a daily basis. The UK youth work tradition shares the social pedagogical values of social learning. Its tradition of direct work with children and families is attractive at a time when many social workers have only limited direct contact. Whether social pedagogues would be collaborators with social workers or competitors to them is a subject of debate. There are those who would like to see existing social workers freed to spend more time in this kind of direct work with children and communities.

In Chapter 4 we will explore social work's relationship to another close neighbour, social care.

IN CONCLUSION

In this chapter we have explored social work's roots and examined some of the major influences that have shaped modern social work. The chapter has aimed to convey the complex nature of social work and the ways in which it is 'contested' – that is, there are often conflcting views of what it is or what it should be. At this stage you might like to turn to pages 115–16 to read about a typical week in social work to get a flavour of social work in practice (not that there is a 'typical' week!). Alternatively, if you would enjoy reading a vision of how social work could look in the future, turn to pages 189–93 (Chapter 7).

FURTHER READING

C.R. Attlee, *The Social Worker*, London: G. Bell and Sons, 1920. (Now a Nabu Public Domain Reprint).

Clement Attlee wrote *The Social Worker* twenty-five years before he became British Prime Minister. It was the first in a series (perhaps the first ever social work book series) which Attlee edited; the other titles were *The Boy*, *The Mother and the Infant*, *The Girl* and *The Worker and the State*. The series was sponsored through Indian philanthropy – the Ratan Tata Department of Social Science at the University of London.

The Social Worker gives a fascinating insight into the state of social work a century ago and the fundamental issues are surprisingly current.

S. Hering and B. Walldijk (eds), *History of Social Work in Europe (1900–1960): Female Pioneers and Their Influence on the Development of International Social Organisations*, Germany: Leske and Budrik, 2003.
An excellent account of the lives of women who pioneered social work in its early years in Europe.

M. Payne, *The Origins of Social Work; Continuity and Change*, Basingstoke: Palgrave Macmillan, 2005.
This book traces the development of social work from its nineteenth-century roots to its current manifestation.

B. Sheldon and G. Macdonald, *A Textbook of Social Work*, London: Routledge, 2009.
A good text; in particular, the first chapter of this book gives an excellent concise history of social work.

N. Thompson, *Understanding Social Work: Preparing for Practice*, Basingstoke: Macmillan, 2000.
Sets social work in its wider context and provides a good overview of the nature, purpose and focus of social work.

E. Younghusband, *The Newest Profession: A Short History of Social Work*, Sutton: Community Care/IPC Business Press, 1981.
A brief account of the history of social work, with a primarily English focus, by the grand dame of British social work. It includes photographs of early social work in action. My acknowledgements to Eileen Younghusband's text for some of the insights in this chapter.

Case Con: a revolutionary magazine for social workers.
Published by British social workers in the UK in the 1970s; if you have access to a successor organisation to a Social Services Department you might find back copies in its library.

SOME RELATED WEBLINKS

www.aaswg.org/standards-social-work-practice-with-groups has a code for standards in groupwork practice.
www.alice-salomon-archiv.de/english/start.html Information about Alice Salomon.

www.basw.co.uk/about/code-of-ethics/ and *www.socialworkers.org/pubs/code/default.asp* provide examples of Codes of Ethics. The British Association of Social Workers was founded in 1970 and its membership in 2011 was 13,000.

www.guardian.co.uk/society/2010/nov/11/social-work-interviews-archive Video interviews with social workers.

www.nasufoundation.org/pioneers/default.asp for information about US social work pioneers. The National Association of Social Workers (US) was established in 1955 and is the largest membership organisation of professional social workers in the world, with 145,000 members in 2011.

www.toynbeehall.org.uk Information about Toynbee Hall.

REFERENCES

Biestek, F.P. (1957), *The Casework Relationship*, Chicago: Loyola University Press.

Gentleman, A. 'Benefit fraud: Spies in the welfare war', *The Guardian*, G2, 1/2/11: 6–11.

Hoggart, S. 'Simon Hoggart's week', *The Guardian*, 10/2/11.

2

HARRIDAN OR HEROINE
THE PUBLIC FACE OF SOCIAL WORK

Stereotypes are inescapable. The popular press in particular likes to present its stories as simple allegories, stripped of the complications of real life. To do this successfully and repeatedly there is a need for a public stock of images that can be recognised without too much effort, rather like the figures in children's fairy tales. Some professions, like the law and medicine, have acquired a wide stock of stereotypes to draw from and provide a range of possibilities from which to construct a story.

Social work has just two basic stereotypes: the wicked witch, turning up to steal your children or offering the promise of an apple (poisoned); and the knight in shining armour, come to the rescue. Wicked witches sell more newspapers.

In this chapter we explore social work's public presence and its response to its representation.

PUBLIC IMAGE

Advertising campaigns to recruit to a profession tell us much about how it is seen. In the UK a campaign to recruit teachers used the slogan 'no-one forgets their teacher'. Famous people gave testimony to how a teacher inspired them to their current success. Soldiers are seen as active team players. The police use their personal skills to defuse tricky situations. Lawyers, doctors and accountants are all too well-paid to need advertising campaigns, though it would be interesting to create slogans for them.

A recruitment crisis in British social work inspired government media campaigns. The print campaign was composed of a series of stories told via ten or so collages. For instance, one told the story of an abused child who is unable to express himself until helped by a social worker through play. The final paragraph in each advert read 'people can be fascinating, mystifying, rewarding, social work is work with people, it's that simple and that complicated'. The strapline was 'Social work – it's all about people.' Unlike the action man army ads and the straightforward hero teachers, the social work campaign tried to convey the subtleties and dilemmas of social work.

No-one forgets a teacher, but who knows what a social worker does? There is poor recognition of social work because few experience it directly and, to some degree, there is a failure by the profession to articulate itself. This is a hard task because there are many views within the profession about what social work is or should be, as we explored in the previous chapter.

HARRIDAN *AND* HEROINE

The title of this chapter, 'Harridan or heroine', is not posed as a question because these two opposites sit side by side in the public consciousness. We see the harridan in full colour at the time of a child murder and the subsequent public inquiry. It would be unusual for a social worker not to be one of the professionals involved in such a situation so social work is often implicated; and social work has been unable to prevent it, whether or not it is reasonable to expect that it could have.

We will explore later how the dynamics of blame feed into the image of the social worker as harridan. Stories of social workers neglecting to intervene where spectators think they should, which would lead to the removal of children from their families, nestle with stories of social workers failing to leave children be and snatching them needlessly. Different conclusions can be drawn from this 'damned if you do, damned if you don't' situation: that social work is rife with incompetence; that these kinds of situation are extremely complicated; that it is hard for spectators to know the full situation.

The social worker as heroine is not so fashionable. There are specific awards that celebrate exceptional if not heroic practice, such as the Social Worker of the Year award. In 2011, social worker Margaret Humphreys received honours in the UK and Australia to mark her campaign for the rights of children from Britain sent to live in other countries without the knowledge and consent of their parents. The story was dramatised in the film *Oranges and Sunshine*.

HUMOUR

If government-sponsored campaigns illustrate the official line on social work, the jokes circulating in the social media are an insight into the unofficial take. Certainly, the public's confused relationship with social work is present in this humour.

Q: What's the difference between a social worker and a pit bull terrier?
A: There's always a chance you'll get your children back from the terrier.

Q: What is the difference between God and a social worker?
A: God doesn't pretend to be a social worker.

A social worker asks a colleague: 'What time is it?' The other one answers: 'Sorry, don't know, I have no watch.' The first one: 'Never mind! The main thing is that we talked about it.'

Q: How many social workers does it take to change a light bulb?
A: None. They set up a team to write a paper on coping with darkness.

Two social workers were walking through a rough part of the city in the evening. They heard moans and muted cries for help from a back lane. Upon investigation, they found a semi-conscious man in a pool of blood. 'Help me, I've been mugged and viciously beaten,' he pleaded. The two social workers turned and walked away. One remarked to her colleague: 'You know the person that did this really needs help.'

What is curious is the mix of all-powerful imagery, illustrated by the first two jokes, and complete ineffectualness, mocked in the others. The fourth casts social workers as unassertive champions of the status quo, for all their supposed radical ideology; and the fifth as very out of kilter with the mainstream.

Though not specifically humorous, other clues about the public image of social work come via the signing for 'social worker' in the deaf community. In fact, this varies between communities, reflecting the different images of the profession. In some deaf dialects the signing indicates a tie (a stuffy official) and in others it is hands behind the head, elbows stretched out, indicating laid back.

BLAME AND THE PUBLIC INQUIRY

The psychology of blame is well established: the wish to understand why something has gone wrong gets enmeshed with the less attractive desire to see someone punished and the even less edifying urge to pin that punishment on the person or group least able to fight back. Blame is more likely to stick to someone who is vulnerable and therefore cannot shake it off, and once it has stuck to someone else we can feel relieved it is not attached to us. There are times when blame is absolutely the correct response, too.

Social workers work with exactly those people who are the most vulnerable and, by association, the profession is liable to attract disproportionate blame and punishment. If social work is doing its job it is making sure the rest of the community knows what it would rather ignore. This might explain why blame is particularly attached to social workers even when doctors and the police are implicated to the same degree or more. A valuable service that social workers can perform is to stand up to the culture of blame in their organisations and in their direct work with service users and the community at large.

The hidden and potential costs of the blame culture are considerable. The Laming report that followed a child murder in 2003 had no less than 58 recommendations and meeting just one of these was independently priced at £116m. The costs of increased referrals following the publicity from the murder are also considerable.

PUBLIC AWARENESS

'What do you do?' is a common enough question at social gatherings, and the reaction to the answer 'social work' is as good a guide as any to public perceptions. It varies from sympathy to conversation-stopping to occasional hostility. (Attlee reported the common view of social workers in 1920 as 'elderly spinsters and men with no settled occupation'!)

The relatively private nature of social work and the fact that it is not a universal experience means that most people's contact, such as it is, comes through the public media. As noted, social work is not depicted in television dramas or soap operas in the way of law and medicine, so it is likely that it is the print media that provide the bulk of any awareness. The high-profile nature of child death cases is likely to skew the public's perception towards social work as primarily concerned with child protection (and failing it).

Occasionally a high-profile figure speaks out about social work. Lord Adonis (a Labour peer in the UK) has spoken publicly about his life in care and about the very positive experience he had of social work. Michael Gove, Education Secretary in the UK Coalition government, has voiced his positive experiences of adoption, if not social work in particular. The pool of celebrities or public figures speaking positively about their social workers will never be as great as those lauding their teachers, but when it happens it is very valuable for social work and influences public attitudes.

Public awareness is exceptionally important because much of the success of social work is affected by the way the public participates in the social realm; for instance, how much engagement there is in the protection of children rather than a reliance on official surveillance by professionals.

PUBLIC SERVICE

Although social work pre-dates the great welfare reforms of the mid-twentieth century, it was big government that provided the boom times, reinforced in the 1960s by the educational expansion that created many new training courses, and in the 1970s by the amalgamation of what were the fragments of social work into powerful social services departments staffed and led by social workers. It is an irony that spending on social work and social care in the UK increased by the greatest proportion during the ministry of Keith Joseph, a politician whose values were the polar opposite to social work.

All public professions benefited from big government, but none more than social work. It is no coincidence that institutions that hate the public realm, such as the UK newspaper the *Daily Mail*, hold social workers in particular contempt. It is not just that the public sector employs large numbers of social workers, certainly in the UK, but that the social work profession prizes the *notion* of public service.

PUBLIC, PRIVATE AND THIRD WAYS

Spending in the public realm returned in the UK during the Labour governments of 1997–2010, but it came with strings attached in the form of targets, government micromanagement and no lessening in the upward sweep of public expectations. Public service furnishes an endless supply of news headlines, mainly its supposed shortcomings, with health, education and crime statistics replacing previous obsessions with private sector failings in the balance of trade and the incompetence of industrial management.

This particular climate change is difficult for social work because of its close association with all that public service symbolises: a commitment to service, funded by the common weal, free of corruption and trusting of professional judgement. The critical question is whether these values can be maintained in a service driven by the profit motive. Examples of the latter, such as the US healthcare system, make many professionals highly sceptical about the possibility of maintaining a public service ethos in a private sector environment.

One response is to consider 'third ways', the possibility of combining public service values with private sector enterprise. New independent social work practices, sometimes called social enterprises or mutuals, are being piloted to test whether there is a third way (or 'fourth way', as the term 'third way' is already seen as tarnished). The fears of those opposed to any move away from public service are, first, the lack of democratic accountability and, second, the vulnerability of these small independent units to bigger commercial fish once they have proved their worth. There is further discussion on pages 120–1.

CUTS

The public sector and, indirectly, much of the not-for-profit sector rely on government finance and have long been prey to changing fiscal and ideological circumstances. A survey of 119 UK social care charities in early 2011 found that two-thirds had had their funding cut from local government councils, more especially the smaller organisations (reported in *Community Care*, 13/1/11: 4). The banking crisis of 2007–8 saw a massive transfer of wealth to the financial sector in the form of bailouts from state treasuries. UK local authorities receiving less public money have limited choices: providing services to fewer people, charging more for services or raising income through increased local taxes. Some believe that redesigning services can make savings but more often this requires initial additional investment before any possible savings are likely to materialise. Demographic changes alone mean that maintaining current services requires an additional one per cent spending per year.

Social work is especially vulnerable at times of cuts because it has a relatively powerless constituency. Education and health provided slogans in recent UK parliamentary elections because there are large sections of the country that use and rely on these services. It brings a smile to the face to think of any political party launching its campaign with a rallying call of 'Social work! Social work! Social work!' ('Education! Education! Education!' was New Labour's slogan in the 1997 UK General Election).

Although the terms of the debate are couched in notions of fairness, in fact cuts to public services invariably affect poor and vulnerable people most. Just one example of this is the impact on the chances of children leaving public care going to university, with the combination of increased university fees and reduced local councils' budgets. Given the unfair impact on marginalised people, it is to be expected that social work mobilises in opposition to these policies; however, there is a tradition of political neutrality in public service, so this creates a tension. However, social work values must lead social workers to speak out when they see injustice and circumstances that worsen the conditions of the people with whom they work.

MEDIA

Research conducted in the late 1980s found that only two of ninety-eight separate UK national news stories with a significant social work component were positive (reported in *Community Care*, 24/3/11: 18). It is useful to remind ourselves of this historical perspective if we view present times as in any way unusual.

PRESS

The press reflects, perhaps helps create, the polarised image of social work that has been discussed in this chapter. The newsprint media include a wide variety of opinion, certainly in the UK, with some papers reliably hostile to the public realm and others less so, even if only to offer sympathy: 'Social workers have been given an impossible job; you have to be mad, desperate or heroic to want to be one' (Madeleine Bunting in the *Guardian*, 22/3/10). Pundits on welfare issues, sometimes referred to as 'welfare insiders', and specialist journalists often attempt to counter the general hostility. the *Guardian*, a national UK newspaper, had just three social policy reporters in the 1960s, a number that grew to thirty by the mid-noughties.

There is no specific consequence to the general media hostility but the regular drip, drip of negative press probably erodes public confidence which, in turn, creates defensiveness. An example is the wariness of providing public funding for sex services (see page 89), even if this might be the right thing to do, because of the likely news stories. Caution about the possible presentation of any service is sensible, but there is a greater need for robust social work press agents, for individual social workers to learn about public communication and for changes in the 'no comment' policies that tie practitioners' hands. We will consider possible strategies for social work later in the chapter.

TV, RADIO AND FILM

Given the human interest and drama inherent in the world of social work it is surprising that it is so little represented in television and film. I have an early recollection of *Probation Officer*, a weekly British television programme, but this was the exception. The only regular comic strip that depicts social work that I know of is Harry Venning's *Clare in the Community*, which appears in the UK weekly *Community Care* and made the transition to a comedy series on BBC radio, more as a sitcom than a commentary on social work. Social workers make occasional cameo appearances in well-established soap operas like *Coronation Street*, but the treatment of social work in popular television reflects the public's general ignorance of what social workers do.

In-depth presentations of social work are limited to occasional documentary series, such as fly-on-the-wall programmes that follow social workers through their working week. However, there are plenty of films that depict situations of great relevance to social work. *Precious*, a 2009 film about an obese, HIV-positive teenager who is made pregnant twice by her father, does feature a rather downtrodden social worker.

References to social work in popular culture can be entertaining. In the 'Gee, Officer Krupke' number from *West Side Story* it is the social worker who takes the hard line. Diagnosed as 'sociologically sick', the juvenile delinquent is referred to a social worker who concludes that, 'deep down inside him, he's no good!'

SOCIAL MEDIA

The impact on social work of social networks such as Twitter and Facebook and professional ones like LinkedIn is still formative. Social workers help pick up the pieces from the fallout of phenomena like internet bullying and practitioners themselves can find themselves the subjects of internet harassment. The internet allows grievances to be aired but often not very responsibly. Practitioners who complain about their managers online need to be aware that this is likely to be construed as unprofessional behaviour and that care should be taken with the way social work is represented through online social networking.

The huge challenge of the internet is the fact that it is unregulated, so the usual boundaries of confidentiality, privacy and responsibility are blurred. The possibility of posting comments about others whilst hiding behind an anonymous online identity does not encourage ownership of these comments, nor restraint. On the other hand, there is tremendous potential to enable isolated people to find others and for people who have lived lives that are physically or emotionally restricted to find expression. Thus far the headlines are more concerned with celebrity lives and the affairs of footballers and it is hard to predict what the ultimate fallout for social work will be, and whether it offers opportunities to promote social work positively.

POLITICS

As public servants, there are some expectations of political neutrality on social workers, certainly in the UK (in the US many social workers run for public office and openly work for political campaigns). On the other hand, social workers' codes of practice and value system require them to combat social injustice and work towards social inclusiveness. These are highly politicised notions, reflecting the political environment in which social work operates. All professions work in this context; the work of medical staff and teachers is profoundly affected by levels of health equality and educational inclusion. However, social work is perhaps the most politicised of professions because, in addition to this general context, social work *is* specifically about working with the social: the clue is in the job title.

In the British political tradition, the weekly surgery that each Member of Parliament holds in their constituency is not dissimilar to community social work. Indeed, an MP discussing the importance of local engagement such as their weekly surgeries remarked, 'Yes, I do social work' (quoted in *Community Care*, 6/5/10).

PARTY POLITICS

Political parties develop their own narratives, such as the UK Conservative Party's 'Broken Britain' and the way it can be mended via the 'Big Society'. These narratives have implications for social work and the profession needs to be able to convey its response to the wider public in the way that the medical and nursing professions have voiced their opposition to the 'reforms' of the National Health Service.

Social work might be a politicised profession regularly in the public glare, but it is rare to see British party politicians rubbing shoulders with social workers, such as being photographed with them or reports of politicians' visits to social workers' places of work. Regular contact with elected politicians is more common in the US, for instance. The social worker as public servant means that few social workers in the UK engage on a regular basis with elected politicians (whether at council or parliamentary level), and this is a loss. In the twenty years I worked as a social worker we were never visited by a Member of Parliament, though I did have regular contact with local councillors. Very few MPs have social work backgrounds, either as qualified social workers or as people who use social work services; teaching, business, law and professional political organisers predominate.

Traditionally, social work has been associated with parties of the left, but we should not forget that the welfare state, established in the UK by the 1945–51 Labour governments, was maintained by subsequent Conservative governments; and that the fragmentation and privatisation of the public realm that began with the Conservative governments of the 1980s continued under New Labour.

As we saw in the first chapter, social work has many roots and these can find expression in different party political affiliations. The radical strain of social work, with its belief in community and collectivist solutions, is drawn more naturally to parties of the left; but there is a conservative social work that is based on a celebration of the individual, freedom from bureaucracy and regulation, and a belief in the primacy of personal change (sometimes springing from religious belief) that lends itself also to liberal and moderate conservative political positions. Marxist priests and radical psychoanalysts reveal the possibilities for seemingly different beliefs and perspectives to find a home together, and party political allegiance is not always predictable.

GRANDSTANDING

Social work is no exception to the easy-win tactic in party politics. An example is the call for social workers to stop waiting for 'perfect' ethnic matches in adoptions, and the accusation that they are delaying placements. In fact this guidance is already in place and operating; what causes most delay is lack of resources for post-adoption care and other complex systemic delays, all of which are much harder to resolve than an easy accusation of political correctness.

Grandstanding is characterised by aggressive pillorying of agencies and individuals followed by public inquiries that make ever more detailed recommendations and central government diktats with complex prescriptions ostensibly to prevent a recurrence; until the next recurrence, when the cycle begins again. This pushes the point of responsibility down the line, so that when the next scandal occurs it cannot be claimed that it was through lack of guidance and, therefore, it was the fault of the social workers who did not follow that guidance.

SOCIAL WORK RESPONSES

Does social work believe that the mass media is unimportant, or has it given up trying to influence it, or does it not have the skills and opportunities to do so? The answer is probably some combination of all three. Certainly, communication with and via mass media is not taught on social work courses in the UK, though public presentation is a feature of US courses. Social workers' hands are tied by those 54 per cent of UK councils which ban them from speaking to the media (*Community Care*, 4/3/10). Perhaps links between courses in social work and journalism might be a better priority for interprofessionalism than the ubiquitous links to nursing?

Child murder puts social work under the hottest spotlight and requires the most regular response. In the UK, the names of Maria Colwell, Tyra Henry, Jasmine Beckford, Victoria Climbié and Peter Connelly tell a similar story over four decades. This fact is a telling one, a reminder that child murder is highly unusual yet recurring. Rates of child murder are steady over the decades and across Western countries. Again, this suggests that we may be at a point where no further reorganisation of services and review of training is likely to have an impact. This is a difficult assertion for the profession and for politicians because of the fear that it is a message that the public is not yet grown up enough to hear. How to present this case without appearing callous and uncaring about those children who do lose their lives? Yet the disruption caused by additional guidance with no accompanying resources is likely to put more children at risk.

There are two main issues, then, that social work must consider in terms of its public face. The first is how to develop public awareness of what social work does, whether this is good, bad or indifferent. In the ad man's jargon, social work has very poor brand recognition. It is difficult for someone to want to be a social worker when they do not know what one is. The second question follows on from the first: once the public recognises what the profession is, how can social work messages be promoted positively?

CAMPAIGNS

The UK government campaign noted earlier to increase awareness of social work did generate interest, and recruitment to social work training courses turned the corner, though the cynics noted that the £2m campaign for social work was outspent threefold by the £6m campaign to recruit for the police. Police work and teaching had additional television and cinema slots.

In 2009, the UK government invested a further £11m in recruitment campaigns and at least £28m in what was termed the social work reform programme. Trade journals like *Community Care* launched a campaign called 'Reclaim Social Work' and invited newly elected MPs to spend a day with social workers, to raise political awareness of social work. The College of Social Work (see later) launched a 'Speak up for Social Work' campaign. It is too soon to judge the impact of these campaigns and resources, but they do indicate that any talk of social work's demise is premature. It is worth remembering that it is now over thirty years since the publication of a book with the infamous title, *Can Social Work Survive?* The lead author was a doctor.

The dilemma about how to respond to media hostility was brought into sharp relief by the inclusion in a UK government-appointed Social Work Task Force of an 'agony aunt' from *The Sun*, a newspaper which is a regular critic of social work. Hostility was the predictable reaction. However, there is a defensible argument that it is better to implicate these forces by inclusion; indeed, this same agony aunt later argued forcibly for the most vulnerable people to escape the cuts of the incoming Coalition government.

COLLEGE OF SOCIAL WORK

Many professions have their own independent professional bodies such as the British Medical Association and the College of Nursing. An independent College of Social Work is being established in England. It will be owned by the profession and the intention is that it will be a strong national voice and provide leadership 'to stand up for social work'. It is charged with defining the values and purpose of social work, tasks one might have hoped did not need to be revisited, but an indication of how contested these have been historically, as we explored in the previous chapter.

The future will see more changes to social work education (possibly moving to a four-year degree in England), the launch of a UK career structure and a compulsory assessed first year of practice.

A figurehead Chief Social Worker is proposed, which would provide the general public with a 'Social Work Tsar' to relate to and, it is to be hoped, to begin to like and trust.

WHISTLEBLOWING

We have been considering broad responses to promote social work's public image, but at an individual level it is also important for social workers to stand up for their profession, especially when they witness unprofessional behaviour and policies. A social worker's professional duty is to draw attention to situations where standards of practice are compromised, but the obstacles to blowing the whistle on poor practice should not be underestimated. Lack of support from colleagues and managers, misguided loyalty to the organisation, uncertainty over the facts and fear of the consequences can all silence an unassertive professional. Will there be a 'blowback', when the failings identified by the whistleblower are seen as their own shortcomings rather than the agency's?

The most common reason for not exposing unprofessional practices is the strength of local culture. If all about you seem to accept what is going on, it takes particular courage and confidence to stick to your guns. The effect of local culture has been found to be exceptionally strong in the police service, but it is undoubtedly a factor in social work, too.

In contrast to the general hostility described so far in this chapter, we should note that the media can play a positive role in exposing poor practice and wrongdoings in social work.

THEMES

EMOTIONAL INVOLVEMENT, STRESS AND BURNOUT

The response to difficult, highly charged situations varies from person to person. One response is to see emotions as in need of control and reason as the antidote to panic. The need to control and rationalise is sometimes referred to as a techno-rational approach and it lies behind the tidal wave of guidance, forms and regulations that are imposed to try to exert control.

In fact, emotional involvement in social work is not just impossible to avoid, but necessary. Balancing emotional engagement with professional detachment is one the most challenging elements of social work and every social worker gets it wrong from time to time. What is important is to know what to do when it does go wrong, to recover the situation and to be able to discuss the experience with a professional supervisor. If these elements are not present the consequences can be levels of stress that lead to burnout. What any social worker hopes to avoid is having a foster parent comment that they 'crackle with stress, like static off nylon tights' (*Guardian Weekend*, 27/11/10: 19). Social worker overload affects the quality of decision-making and puts service users at risk.

One aspect of burnout is compassion fatigue in which close and regular proximity to traumatic events has the potential to traumatise social workers. Groupwork has been found to be effective to support social workers at risk of this kind of burnout. Critical incident debriefing is a way to work through the aftermath of traumatic events experienced through work and is especially important for social workers involved in high-profile emergencies.

Because of the traumatic nature of some of the work, social workers should make sure they have self-care time, some form of regular 'healing' time each week. This will mean different things to different people. For me it was a regular swim session taken with a few colleagues. We each made sure it went in our diaries like a regular appointment, so we knew we would be waiting for one another. This prevented any temptation to skip.

TABOOS

Social work frequently works head on with social taboos. There are many examples, but let us consider dementia and sexual behaviour:

> Responses to the news that two residents suffering from dementia are engaged in sexual relations are likely to include concern, shock, possibly outrage. Older men, in particular, are likely to be judged as predatory by the wider public.
>
> Social workers must carefully consider the competing arguments, in this case between the expression of human needs and the protection of defenceless people. It is not unusual for new relationships to form in

residential care. Older people still have sexual needs, and affection and intimacy contribute to a feeling of well-being. The social work response to taboo issues of this kind is, first, not to react on the basis of one's own preferences, but carefully to consider the facts of the situation. For instance, do the parties have the mental capacity to consent to sexual relations? Can they express their own views, if only at certain more lucid times? Do they recognise and remember the person with whom they are having the relationship? What effect does the relationship seem to be having on the partners (do they seem generally more content or more agitated)? Decisions must be made in the partners' own best interests and not on the basis of moralising.

How it will look if the mass media get their hands on the story is not the best way to make these kinds of sensitive, highly tuned decisions. Public prurience in taboo topics is, of course, a reality and social work will always have a difficult job to explain the subtleties of complex social and personal situations.

LANGUAGE

The language of social work has changed over the years and one of the biggest changes is indicated in the title of the next chapter (i.e. the term for the people who use social work). The language of yesteryear can strike us as crass and judgemental: Attlee uses 'morally defective', a prevailing term at the time of his 1920 book, *The Social Worker*. We need to see these descriptions in the context of their time and not dismiss them out of hand simply because they depart from current convention.

JARGON

It is natural for a professional community to develop its own shorthand, but it has a responsibility to maintain multilingual skills so that it can revert to general English when speaking with others. Service users can often find themselves excluded on the basis of the language that social workers choose to use. Social work has not been immune to the language of business management and cliché:

Market conditions in social care will see an improved flow of service delivery opportunities to end-users and participant stakeholders, with the social work agenda creating synergies between social care governance and choice-driven, modernised, point-of-access services.

The growth of acronyms rather than single words or phrases is also notable in social work, sometimes with amusing results. I have always known the PLO to be the Palestine Liberation Organisation but in British social work it became a Practice Learning Opportunity ('placement' to the rest of the world). Much jargon is not recognised as such. The business term *stakeholders* has taken complete hold of UK social work. 'Vulnerable' is a perfectly ordinary English word but its frequent use, as in 'vulnerable people', attaches the situation to the person, so that rather than being a situation (which is external and temporary) it becomes a condition (which is personal and permanent). It is reasonable to suppose that this affects the thinking of those who perceive others as vulnerable. Whilst the contraction of 'people currently in a vulnerable situation' to 'vulnerable people' is understandable, there is a price to pay in the distortion in meaning. There are parallels with a previous social work generation's talk of 'problem families': they were families with problems and the casual contraction of the language affected the way in which professionals and the wider community perceived them.

Academic and professional language can be pompous. An example is the way 'utilise' is overwhelming the simpler 'use'. There is no sentence in which utilise cannot be replaced by use and retain exactly its meaning. Utilise is an example of leverage (to use more jargon); that is, trying to make the meaning seem more substantial than it is. Clumsy compound verbs are common, as in 'Jordan's mother was risk-assessed.'

By and large, changes in social work language have tended to come from outside social work, especially business management, and this has not helped the profession to communicate with the wider public. Changes in terms obscure the historical lineage, because the name change suggests a real change when, often, there is none. An example of this is the way child protection has become child safeguarding; it is difficult to know why there are two terms for the same thing. 'Abuse' and 'neglect' are out of fashion, yet they are common words that are easily understood by the public.

POLITICAL CORRECTNESS

The term *political correctness* has undergone changes. Initially it denoted language and behaviours that minimise possible offence on the basis of gender, race and ethnicity, etc., but it was usurped by the political right as a pejorative term denoting Stalinist orthodoxy and the term politically *in*correct has become a badge of self-praise.

Political correctness is significant because of its strong association in the public mind with social work. The use of the term as a slogan is usually a substitute for careful reasoning. 'Political correctness slowing down adoptions says children's minister' was a headline relating to the complex issue of whether children should be placed with families of the same race as themselves. The ethical and practical considerations, the pros and cons, are all very complicated, the evidence base is far from clear and there are conflicting individual testimonials; so the slogan 'political correctness' is being used to appeal to prejudices and to cut through any careful and difficult weighing of the arguments. Multiculturalism is another term that is becoming a slogan, again used to pre-empt any reasoned argument.

Turns of phrase are significant: 'people with personality disorder' is not the same as 'personality-disordered individual'. The former is more respectful and the latter is an example of 'labelling'. The language used is likely to reflect the attitudes of the speaker and experience suggests that changing language can change attitudes. Proper sensitivity to language to ensure that it is respectful and non-judgemental is true to social work's humanist roots. Attacks on this are also assaults on the value base of social work; hyperbole is used to rubbish what is an admirable and essential element of social work.

IN CONCLUSION

In this chapter we have explored public perceptions of social work and, in particular, its treatment in the public media. A key issue is the fact that social work is not a universal service and, therefore, many people have not experienced it directly, so media representations may provide their only information. Hostility to public service in general is especially strong in sections of the print media, which often encourage a blame culture. Social work needs to become politically savvy and more proactive in campaigning and presenting itself to the wider world. It is important to avoid jargon and business terminology: language is important and should be respectful of people and their circumstances.

FURTHER READING

M. Dean, *Democracy Under Attack – How the Media Distort Policy and Politics*, Bristol: Policy Press, 2011.
The author is a long-standing specialist journalist in social care and founding editor of *The Guardian*'s 'Society' section. The book explores the impact of the media, not just on social work and social care but on broader democratic processes.

M.L. Freeman and D.P. Valentine, 'Through the eyes of Hollywood: images of social workers in film', *Social Work*, 2004 Apr.; 49[2], pp. 151–56.
This journal article analysed forty-four films spanning the period from 1938 to 1998, with particular attention to the themes of gender, race and class.

N. Stanley and J. Manthorpe (eds), *The Age of the Inquiry: Learning and Blaming in Health and Social Care*, London: Routledge, 2004.
This book presents various perspectives on public inquiries into deaths of children, people with learning disabilities and older people, and insights into the role of the media.

P. Williams, *Precious: A True Story*, London: Bloomsbury, 2010.
This is the story of a black child growing up in a white foster family. It gives a very balanced picture of the pros and cons of interracial fostering and adoption and makes the term 'political correctness' look embarrassingly naive. 'I wish my foster family had said "You're a black girl and that's great" instead of "We don't see you as black – we love you." But, hey, at least they loved me and told me so every day.'

M. Wright, *Be Lucky*, Deptford: Deptford Forum Publishing, 2003.
An example of a book written by an author who was a social worker for twenty years. It is centred on a local community pub and, though it is not specifically about social work, it draws from the author's experiences as a social worker.

SOME RELATED WEBLINKS

www.collegeofsocialwork.org The College of Social Work is an independent organisation to represent and support the social work profession in the UK.
www.communitycare.co.uk/carespace/forums is a UK example of social networking in social work and social care.

www.guardian.co.uk/society/social-care provides current news about social work and social care.

www.helpstartshere.org is an American information site about social work practice for the community at large.

www.scie-socialcareonline.org.uk Social Care Online has reports of UK social care public inquiries.

www.suntimes.btinternet.co.uk/intersite/swjokes.html has more social work humour.

REFERENCES

Bunting, M. 'We have to manage the expectations of child protection, and not turn social workers into figures of contempt', the *Guardian*, 22/3/10.

Community Care (2010), 'In danger of dilution', 6/5/10.

Community Care (2010), 'It's now time to talk', 4/3/10.

Community Care (2011), 'Services and jobs slashed as councils cut grants to voluntary sector', 13/1/11: 4.

Community Care (2011), 'Let's make the right headlines', 24/3/11: 18.

Guardian Weekend (2010), 'Foster carer's diary – March', 27/11/10: 19.

3

CLIENTS OR SERVICE USERS
HOW AND WHY PEOPLE COME INTO CONTACT WITH SOCIAL WORK

In this chapter we will explore the relationship between social workers and the people with whom they work and consider the circumstances that bring them together.

NEITHER UNIVERSAL NOR MAINSTREAM

Most people have not experienced social work first hand, unlike other services such as medicine, teaching and policing. Social work is different; it is not a universal service.

The following figures show the numbers of qualified social workers per 10,000 people in the UK compared to some other professions:

- social workers: 10–15
- teachers: 380
- doctors: 22
- police officers: 20

The figures for the numbers of people who come into contact with these respective services are not available but we can assume that experience of social work is least common. Not only are the numbers of people who experience social work small relative to other public services, but most of these people are at the margins of society. They are unlikely to be well-connected or to move on to powerful positions in government or commerce; their voices are often unheard and frequently represent sections of the community that are outside the norm. Social work is neither a mainstream nor a universal service. Indeed, it is often seen as stigmatising and undesirable.

CLIENTS

The term client has long been used to describe the people who use social work services. 'Client' was seen as a way of professionalising the relationship between social workers and the people with whom they worked: lawyers have clients, public relations and media people have client accounts. 'Patient' was seen as too medicalised, though some medical social workers did speak of patients, adopting the language of their colleagues.

There are flaws with 'client'. First, there are pejorative associations. Client states, for instance, are inferior nations that are in hock to more powerful ones. Lawyers might have clients, but so do sex workers. Client also implies a paying relationship that is usually absent in social work. In all other circumstances, clients hire and fire the professional in question, but this is far from the case with social workers. In other professions clients are there in a voluntary capacity, whereas there are many occasions when social work clients would prefer not to be clients, as we will explore later. It would be strange to call people charged for offences by the police as 'clients' of the police service.

Terms have a shelf-life. 'Social security' was initially coined as a precise description of its purpose and what could be more admirable than a notion of social security? Over time the coinage becomes debased by the reality, so that a new descriptor such as 'income support' is found necessary, until this in turn is considered to need polishing. 'Client' has experienced this same effect.

In some English-speaking countries, notably the United Kingdom, the clients themselves became more active in defining or redefining their status and 'client' did not match their vision of this new status. The term gives off a whiff of deference or subservience that is no longer seen to fit a notion of empowerment and self-direction. In the UK the term 'service user' has eclipsed client.

Doctors have patients and teachers have students and they always have had. These terms do not have a shelf-life. Yet social work, a relatively young profession, cannot settle comfortably on a word to describe the people with whom it works, for service user is not universally welcomed and 'client' is still prevalent in some parts of the world, such as the US. Other terms, such as 'customer', are sometimes used; and certain groups, such as people with learning difficulties, might choose to describe themselves as 'self-advocates'. As we learned in the previous chapters, social work is a highly contested profession (that is, people have very different ideas about what it is or should be) and it is fitting that the word used to describe the people who use social work is also contested.

In this book we shall follow British social work convention and, by and large, use the term 'service user'. The simple term 'user' is sometimes employed, but the specific association of 'user' with drug user means that it is generally less popular than 'service user'.

WHO BECOMES A SERVICE USER AND HOW?

Since social work is neither a universal nor a mainstream service what, then, connects the people who use social work? In some respects the answer is very little other than the 'social work' and we will learn more about what this social work is in the next chapter. What service users have in common is that they are usually experiencing troubles or they are in trouble, but the nature of these troubles varies enormously.

LIFE COURSE

There are many ways in which we could approach the question 'who becomes a service user?' – but let's take the life course as a way of charting contact with social work.

Before life is even born, a woman might seek social work advice concerning a possible abortion or adoption for her child. Prospective adoptive parents will have contact with a social worker during the period of assessment for suitability and once any child is placed with them. At birth, in some circumstances, a mother might have her baby removed by a social worker, with or without her consent. A mother whose child is born prematurely might seek help and information from hospital-based social work. Following birth, a mother suffering from post-puerperal psychosis might have contact with a social worker, or perhaps as a mother with post-natal depression she will join a group led by a social worker. Very occasionally, the father or partner of someone suffering post-natal depression might join a support group led by a social worker.

Health visitors provide the universal service for infants, but if there are particular social problems in the family or the child has developmental difficulties, social work can help. A schoolchild experiencing problems in school or at home, or both, might receive support from a social worker. These problems might loosely be described as 'social' but could have any combination of emotional, psychological, cognitive and physical aspects. Children who are in foster homes or residential care will experience social work. As a young person grows into adolescence, perhaps he or she gets into trouble with the law and encounters social work in the courts and, subsequently, in a youth offending team.

At any stage in a person's life mental health problems might be experienced, sometimes relatively minor, at other times possibly severe and enduring, and occasionally necessitating compulsory admission to hospital. They will likely become a 'mental health service user'. People with disabilities – physical, sensory (hearing, seeing) or cognitive (intellectual and learning difficulties) – are also likely at some stage to use social work.

People who find themselves homeless, dependent on alcohol or drugs, living with HIV-AIDS, seeking asylum, refugees in a new country, abused by their partner or carer, and subject to any number of other personal and social ills, might find themselves with social work services.

As people age, their independence can become compromised and they might find themselves users of social care services to help support them in their own home. If the problems are particularly difficult, such as dementia, they might encounter social work.

One social ill that I have not mentioned is poverty. Although social problems might lead to, or arise from, poverty, social work in Britain has not had a role in income support in the way that it has in some countries, like Norway. So, being poor does not of itself mean that you will be a service user, though many service users are poor.

The simplest way to describe all of this is 'social problems', though the breadth of these problems is a problem in itself. As we will see in the next chapter, social work finds itself in an interesting place, often between the gaps of the other services or overarching them. Most professions have a particular focus or specialism, but social workers, as the title suggests, lift their eyes to see a cinemascopic view of the people they work with: classically, the *whole person* in their family and their community, the person as a social being in the social world.

However, we will discover in the next chapter that the ways in which social work is organised and social workers are employed have a powerful influence on defining who might become a service user.

In the next pages of this chapter we will consider in a little more detail the various life situations that can bring people into contact with social work. It is important to emphasise that the categories below are not mutually exclusive; a child might suffer poor mental health, for example. However, as we will see in the next chapter, the boundaries erected by the services (children's services, mental health services, etc.) can be barriers for service users with multiple problems.

LOOKING AFTER OTHER PEOPLE'S CHILDREN

Caring for other people's children, whether on a permanent or temporary basis, is demanding and not without controversy. Some cultures accept notions of adoption and fostering more readily than others and the idea of family is fluid in some societies, more rigid in others. Is gender unimportant (as in adoption by a same-sex couple), yet race/ethnicity significant (so that placements should be matched for racial and cultural origins)? Social work is at the heart of adoption and fostering and social workers must be able to navigate the controversies in this field of practice as well as developing the skills to come to a judgement about the likely best needs of the child.

ADOPTION

Adoption is often referred to as 'permanence planning' and it is a response to the need some children have for a permanent family when their own family is unable to care for them, and when it is assessed that, even with help and support, it is unlikely that their own family will be able to provide adequate care.

Adoption rates in the UK are falling. The numbers of children placed for adoption dropped from 2,700 children in 2009 to 2,300 in 2010, a 15 per cent decline. About a quarter of children with an adoptive plan are never successfully matched with an adoptive family and the overall number of final adoption orders in the UK is also falling, from 3,700 in 2006 to 3,200 in 2010. Finding appropriate adoptive parents is, therefore, very important; if all plans reached fruition it would see adoptions rise considerably. Previously, there were targets for adoption numbers and some feel these should be reintroduced to apply political pressure to the system.

Adoption remains controversial because it is such a final step. 'Open adoption', in which there is some formalised contact between the child and its birth parent or parents, is one way in which the finality of adoption can be softened. This principle is now embraced by adoption law in the UK, but not, for instance, in Ireland.

Rates of adoption breakdown are not collected nationally in the UK, but anecdotal evidence perhaps contributes to some reluctance to make adoption orders and to favour alternatives such as special guardianship orders (SGOs), which were created in the Adoption and Children Act 2002 (England and Wales) to keep children in their birth families. In addition, there are concerns about the relative lack of post-adoption support, especially with cuts to budgets.

Social workers are involved in all aspects of the adoption process: recommending children for adoption; vetting adoptive parents; and as Guardians who make recommendations about adoption and prepare reports for the court. They might lead groups for prospective adoptive parents and provide support after an adoption has been granted. There is a trade-off between having sufficient time to make the best decision for a child, but not leaving a child in unstable circumstances with no decision about their future. This is highly skilled social work, requiring judgements that will have a profound effect on a child's life and the lives of the child's birth family and adoptive family.

FOSTERING

Children who cannot be cared for by their own family are sometimes placed with another family, where they are fostered. This is usually considered to be a temporary arrangement whilst more permanent plans are made for the child, perhaps to return to the birth family or to move into more specialised care (such as residential care) or to be placed for adoption.

Foster care is also a possible alternative to custody for young offenders, more especially where the criminal behaviour is seen to be rooted in the young person's family experiences and environment. This kind of 'intensive fostering' includes support from family therapists as well as social workers.

Foster parents receive training and support from social workers and are considered to be colleagues. One foster carer describes her social worker as 'nice but needy', a reminder that assessments are being made in both directions (the *Guardian*, 27/11/10). Opening up your home to a stranger, and one who is likely to be experiencing considerable troubles, is demanding and it is important that everyone is aware of the strengths and limitations of each particular foster family in relation to the possible placement of a foster child. The impact on the foster family's own children should not be underestimated. However, limited numbers of foster placement vacancies mean that decisions are often taken on pragmatic grounds. Other complexities are the need to find and provide education and leisure activities for fostered children and arrangements for them to maintain contact with their birth families.

Apart from the obvious difference between adoption and fostering (permanent and temporary) the financial arrangements also differ, with adoptive parents taking full financial responsibility for their children whilst foster families receive allowances to support their work. These allowances are not abundant: one foster parent calculated it at £2.14 per hour per child (*Guardian Weekend*, 27/11/10: 23). In most cases the foster family and the foster children have their own, different social workers to support them.

Private foster care is a controversial area. Although adoption and fostering is generally highly regulated in the UK compared with the US, it is estimated that there are anything between 10,000–20,000 children in foster care arrangements in the UK that have been made without any social work oversight. Legislation now requires that local authorities are notified. Although some provide good care, the murder of Victoria Climbié in the UK in 2000 whilst in a private fostering arrangement alerts us to the possible dangers and suggests the need for caution about any moves to deregulate fostering.

CHILDREN AND FAMILIES

Social workers play a major part in supporting children in their own families, protecting children in vulnerable situations and working with children who are neglected or abused. They work with children who are still at home and also those who may have been taken into public care, often termed 'looked after' or 'accommodated'. In 2011 there were 65,000 children in care in England, 5,000 more than ten years earlier. The overall cost of looked-after children in care in the UK is estimated at about £2.5bn.

CHILDREN LEAVING CARE

Social workers help children in care prepare for independent life following their eighteenth birthday, providing support as they move out of care. However, most children growing up in their families of birth expect to be able to live with their parents beyond their eighteenth birthday and to return home for periods after that. It is unrealistic to expect children who have grown up in care to achieve independence, however defined, by a specified date and schemes like 'Staying Put' support young people in residential or foster care past the age of 18 (see weblinks at the conclusion of this chapter). This means that young people can make their choices at their own pace and with continuing support.

CHILD CRUELTY

Social work is concerned with the protection of people in vulnerable situations (sometimes called 'safeguarding'), none more so than children and young people at risk of significant harm. It is still not really understood why some adults are cruel to children, though there is often a pattern in which the adult, too, experienced cruelty as a child.

Social work has a role to play in the support of families to prevent abuse, in the detection of cruelty and non-accidental injuries, in the removal of children to safety, and in the prosecution of the people who have perpetrated the abuse. Social workers work with other professionals to fulfill these complex roles in many ways. We will consider social work methods in Chapter 4.

The picture is further complicated when it is children who are cruel to other children. Social work's role is not just to seek to prevent this, but to ask broader social questions, such as why a child murderer elicits more public outrage than an adult murderer. This was particularly illustrated in England by the response to the murder of 2-year-old James Bulger by two 10-year-old children in 1993.

The new technologies mean that abuse can take place online, too. In the UK the Child Exploitation and Online Protection Centre (now amalgamated with the National Crime Agency) investigates these instances and provides both technical and therapeutic support to victims, as well as providing digital evidence to locate and prosecute predators.

Abuse can be physical, sexual and emotional. It can be subtle and not always easy to define. Is obesity a child protection issue, for instance? Should children be removed from parents who make no attempt to address their child's weight?

EARLY INTERVENTION AND PREVENTION WORK

The high profile cases of child abuse should not obscure the considerable amount of time that is spent in preventive work, where social work helps to prevent families getting into more difficult situations. There is research to suggest that early intervention with families can have a considerable impact, though it is always difficult to prove what would have happened if there had not been an intervention. Early intervention is often conceived as a more universal approach than preventive work, especially in early childhood intervention. In many respects cases of long-term chronic neglect can be more challenging than the rarer, higher profile child cruelty.

Resources for preventive work are stretched and the threshold between what might be considered a child protection case and a case where a child is 'in need' is always difficult to determine. The hysterical public and political response at times of high profile child murders diverts already scarce resources away from prevention into protection, even though the statistics show that the rate of child murder remains steady (and is exceptionally low), whatever shape the services take and no matter how many rules and procedures are in place. In a poll, 94 per cent of respondents felt the Chief Executive of the National Society for the Prevention of Cruelty to Children (NSPCC) was right to admit that we may never end child cruelty (*Community Care*, 25/2/10: 14).

Preventive work can be bolstered by 'respite care', in which brief, planned care is provided outside the person's family to provide some relief and refreshment. The plan is always for a return to the family home, and the hope is that all involved will feel the benefit of the change.

COURT WORK AND YOUTH JUSTICE

Social workers work closely with the courts, in particular the family court system. In England Cafcass (Children and Family Court Advisory and Support Service) provides reports to the court and is particularly concerned to represent the child's voice in legal proceedings such as custody of children following divorce. In public law the average length of cases is about 56 weeks and the cost of the family justice system is estimated at £1.6bn a year. The family court system is, therefore, under considerable pressure and there is more emphasis on family mediation and dispute resolution as ways of avoiding court. Social work and the legal profession need to work closely together for these systems to be effective.

The age of criminal responsibility is 10 in England, Wales and Northern Ireland and 12 in Scotland. There is pressure to raise this age to 12 or 14, which would decriminalise children in those age groups. A survey by the Prison Reform Trust showed that half of children in custody live in deprived households of poor housing and the links between criminal behaviour, poverty and deprivation are strong. Social work has a large part to play in supporting children, young people and their families in these circumstances.

Youth Offending Teams are multi-professional teams working with young offenders. There is a mix of individual and groupwork to help offenders to understand what led them to commit an offence, the consequences of their actions for themselves and the victims, and ways in which they can avoid future unlawful activity. Many of the methods used by these teams derive from social work models and social workers are likely to be involved in restorative justice programmes. These focus on the *needs* of all involved (victims, offenders and local communities) rather than punishment. Victims play an active role, which counters their sense of victimhood, and offenders face the responsibility that comes from understanding the consequences of their crimes.

DISABILITIES

Social workers work with people with many different kinds of disability, some associated with increasing age. Social workers help people to remain as independent as they can be in their own homes, often working with occupational therapists to adapt homes in ways which make them safer and more accessible to their inhabitants. They support older people who are moving into residential or nursing care, working closely with any person who is caring for the person (known as a carer).

Accident and illness might mean that a person becomes disabled at a younger age, perhaps even as a child. Social workers work with people across the age range, often providing specialist help, for instance in spinal injury units, providing a wide range of services from counselling and emotional support to practical assistance and liaison between home and hospital.

People with sensory disabilities (blindness, deafness and other visual and hearing impairments) are likely to have specialist support from rehabilitation workers, but social workers might also be involved, especially if the individual is experiencing other difficulties in their life.

There is a wide spectrum of learning disability, from relatively mild (such as some forms of dyslexia) to relatively severe (some forms of autism). A learning disability can have an impact on a person's intellectual, social and motor abilities and, depending on the severity and the circumstances, they might be helped and supported by social work. Past terms for learning disability have been extremely pejorative (such as 'moron' and 'feeble-minded') and indicate the severe discrimination that this group of people has experienced.

In the UK social workers are not directly involved in income support; nevertheless, the numbers of people who receive incapacity benefit or income support who are also users of social work services is large. Given the review of these benefits over the coming years, there is likely to be increased work for social workers called on by claimants seeking their support to maintain their benefits. Cuts to housing benefit and disability living allowances would lead to increased financial difficulties for disabled people in the UK, with consequences for social workers' workloads.

MENTAL HEALTH

Mental health problems are common in the population and the consequences and costs of mental ill-health are far-reaching and considerable. One in six adults in the UK between the ages of 18 and 65 has symptoms of mental illness, of which the most common are depression and anxiety disorders; two per cent are diagnosed with schizophrenia or bipolar (manic/depressive) disorder. Estimates suggest that one in ten children has a mental health problem. Amongst people aged over 65, depression and dementia are the most common mental health issues, with rates of dementia as high as 30 per cent in people aged over 90.

Social workers work with people in a wide range of mental health situations in the community and in institutions. Social work is concerned with the social determinants of mental health; that is, the social causes and social meanings of mental illness. For example, how might the higher rates of schizophrenia and other psychoses amongst black Caribbean and African populations be explained? Similarly, rates of self-harm differ significantly between ethnic groups, with the highest rates amongst black females aged 18–34, yet this group is least likely to gain access to psychiatric care. Studies suggest that many of the social determinants of mental ill-health and mental well-being have their roots in childhood. Certainly, early treatment improves the long-term prognosis for mental illnesses such as psychosis.

As in most other areas of professional social work, mental health work is undertaken by teams that are usually composed of different professions. Social workers have an important role in helping the team understand the social model of health and disability (see Chapter 1) and we will consider social work's specific contribution in Chapter 4.

COMPULSORY ADMISSION TO HOSPITAL

When the mental illness is very severe it can pose dangers to the person and to others. This is especially true when the person is unaware of their problems and not able to understand them. Social workers in the UK are tasked with assessing people for (compulsory) hospital admission under the Mental Health Act (1983, amended 2007). At one time these powers were restricted to a person with a social work qualification (together with a psychiatrist), though legislation has broadened this to an Approved Mental Health Practitioner so that, for instance, mental health nurses can also perform this role.

Social workers might also be Independent Mental Health Advocates, advocating on behalf of a service user where there is a contested or complex assessment of the person's mental health. Determining whether hospital admission is in the person's best interests is complicated and often fraught, especially if the person's mental capacity is impaired, for example by a learning disability.

DRUG AND ALCOHOL MISUSE

There are an estimated 300,000 users of heroin and crack in the UK and a much larger, but difficult to estimate, number of people with alcohol-related problems. Almost 10,000 deaths a year in the UK are directly attributed to alcohol and many more are alcohol-related; for example, nearly half of those who commit murder in Scotland, whose drink status is known, were drunk at the time of the offence.

Although social work has much to offer people who misuse drugs and alcohol, there is also evidence to suggest that there is a knowledge gap, with many social workers unsure of this area of work. In particular, social workers can see their role as ending once a person has been referred to a specialist drug and alcohol action team. Yet the misuse of drugs and alcohol has profound effects on a person's mental health, their ability to care for themselves and their children, and the likelihood that they will commit crimes, most notably to fund their habit. For all these reasons it is important that social workers look out for the possibility of substance misuse and consider what social work has to offer people in these circumstances.

Social work, with its critical social policy perspective, looks deeper than individual treatments. It concerns itself with the effects of drug prohibition policies and the criminalisation of drugs. This brings an understanding that current prohibition policies bring an endless supply of service users to drug treatment services.

REFUGEES, ASYLUM SEEKERS AND TRAVELLERS

A refugee is someone offered protection in accordance with the Refugee Convention 1951 and granted leave to stay, whilst an asylum seeker has asked for protection but has yet to receive a decision. In 2008 there were over 25,000 applications for asylum in the UK, 70 per cent of which were refused at first application.

The social work approach to refugees and asylum seekers is consistent with a human rights perspective. This ensures dignity and respect, not just a sole focus on eligibility and status. So, if a refused asylum seeker is in need of care services but is not eligible, they should be assessed under the Human Rights Act to establish whether it would breach their human rights not to provide services.

Access to services is particularly difficult for people who are new to the country and do not speak or read English, so low take-up of services does not therefore indicate that the services are not needed. It is always good practice to involve service users in the services that are provided, but in work with refugees and asylum seekers this is absolutely critical so that services can accommodate cultural differences. Linking community groups with individual asylum seekers and services is crucial and this networking and co-ordination is a social work skill.

The experiences of migrants before they arrive in the UK are likely to have been traumatic and it is no surprise that they are at high risk of poor mental health and social exclusion. Social work has a potentially very significant role with refugees and asylum seekers, but scarce resources and other priorities have meant that this potential is yet to be developed.

Travellers, also known as Roma or Gypsies, are often described as a marginalised group living outside mainstream society. They are not a small group (one London borough alone has 2,500 travellers) and social work has a role to work with travellers to help them to manage the demands of the wider society and to help the wider society to understand travellers. This requires a community-based practice in which trust can be established over a period of time.

OLDER PEOPLE

Social workers work with older people who need assistance to stay in their own homes. In previous times this would have involved hands-on working, but it is more likely to take the form of care management, in which the social worker co-ordinates a package of care. Increasingly, individuals have control of their own resources ('personalisation' – see page 78), so their call on social work expertise is more about local knowledge of possible services.

Domiciliary, day and residential services might be part of the care package. Domiciliary services bring help (home help) into the person's own home, whilst day care provides opportunities for socialisation and personal care (hairdressing, foot care, etc.). Residential care can be available on a respite basis, that is periodic, planned times in residential care, perhaps to provide intensive care for the older person and some relief for a carer; or permanent residential care, either in a social care home or a nursing home, the latter providing nursing care. There is also specialist care for older people who suffer dementia in homes for elderly mentally infirm people.

Social work plays an important role in supporting individuals and their families through these difficult transitions.

The demands on social work vary from area to area. For example, work with military families and veterans is a significant component of some US-based social work. In countries that have experienced recent civil war and unrest, such as Georgia, work with Internally Displaced Persons (IDPs) is a significant part of the workload.

SERVICE USERS WHO DO NOT WANT TO BE SERVICE USERS

Most people who are interested in becoming social workers are motivated by a desire to help. In training to become social workers they learn about the need to help people find their strengths and build on them and to step into others' shoes in order to understand the world as they do. They develop a critical approach to social policy which casts individuals' actions in a broader, deeper context and highlights the effects of discrimination, oppression and deprivation rather than personal blame or evil.

High levels of empathy and optimism do not necessarily equip social workers to recognise and deal with manipulation and deceit. However, as many case reviews reveal, social workers meet some people who are very skilled at not revealing themselves and who use methods that aim to distract, deceive or intimidate. For example, a service user making aggressive accusations that the social worker's questioning of their parenting is a racist act (see the case inquiry into the death of Khyra Ishaq, 2008).

Police officers have a wide repertoire of possible responses to violence and aggression, but social workers tend to rely on communication skills to defend themselves. The police practice of working in pairs is limited by resources in social work. There are, then, many ways in which social workers are vulnerable and do not have the power that is often ascribed to them.

It is important to retain a sense of balance; high profile cases should not obscure the fact that many people are open to social work help. Most people would prefer not to be in situations where social work is needed or warranted, but initial reluctance can usually turn into active engagement. This makes it all the more difficult for social workers to retain the degree of sceptical distance necessary to recognise cases of 'disguised compliance', when service users say one thing and do another.

SERVICE USERS PROVIDING AND BUYING SOCIAL SERVICES

This chapter has explored who might use social work services and in what circumstances. In recent years there has been a movement to develop services that are *provided* by service users themselves.

A user-led organisation is one that is run and controlled by people who use social services. An early example in the UK was the Independent Living Organisation, which developed in the 1980s to enable disabled people to lead independent lives. Typically, this kind of organisation will provide advocacy and support for other users. 'Shaping Our Lives' is a user-led organisation that places emphasis on the expertise that derives from direct, lived experience (see weblinks at the conclusion of this chapter). One of the terms sometimes used for service users is 'experts by experience'.

Some might go so far as to say that only a service user can really understand another service user. Certainly, the perspective of a service user is different from that of a social worker, though we should remember that some social workers are also users of social services, too. However, growing up in care does not necessarily mean you would make a good social worker, just as growing up in school classrooms could not guarantee that you would be a good teacher. Perhaps the working relationship between service user and social worker is happiest when each respects and understands what the other has to bring, whether this is direct experience or not.

It is hoped that user-led organisations make services more relevant to the people who use them. However, they tend to be small organisations and can find it difficult to compete for resources with larger bodies.

'PERSONALISATION'

Personalisation is a buzz word in social care in the UK. It aims to give individuals more say about what would best meet their needs, including their own personal budgets to spend, and to move away from assessments that are led by professionals such as social workers, and towards self-assessments by service users. Personalisation has long been a core social work value, if not by this name; however, its current manifestation is consumerised and reflects the market approach (i.e. buying and selling services) that dominates.

People who hold their own personal budgets are *consumers* of social services. Indeed, the most expensive 'care package' for a single service user in the UK is thought to be £650,000 ($1m) a year. This came to light when the person moved to a new authority which was required to pick up this bill. Only when service users join forces, for instance when they participate in user-led organisations, might they develop the power to be *commissioners* of social services with more opportunity to shape those services. Then they can hope to prise local authorities out of their perceived role as gatekeepers of how they, the authorities, think individual budgets should be spent. However, 'choice' should mean service users could choose council-managed personal budgets and services, too. Indeed, this might be a case of fixing something that isn't broken, as a survey of service users in 2010 found high levels of satisfaction with existing local authority services, suggesting that there will continue to be a demand for traditional services such as day centres.

Personalisation exposes one of the dilemmas at the heart of social work: how do professional social workers marry their expertise to that of the people with whom they work? The best outcome is when both sets of expertise can come together, with as little procedural burden as possible.

CARERS

The formal social services that employ social workers and social care staff are small compared to the vast numbers of people who are caring for their family, neighbours and friends in an informal, unpaid way. These people are often called carers and there are an estimated six million in the UK.

The situation of informal carers has been increasingly acknowledged and the care they give recognised. In some circumstances, the state provides financial support in recognition of the huge costs that the public finances would bear without this army of unpaid carers, the large majority of whom are women. However, most payments to carers are in the form of one-off payments rather than longer-term financial support. There is a need for individual service users and carers to be able to pool their sources of financial support into a 'family budget'.

The particularly difficult situation of young carers should be noted. A BBC survey in 2010 found that the numbers of young people acting as carers for parents or other relatives in the UK is probably much higher than the 2001 census figures indicated (250,000 rather than 175,000). Although a child caring for a parent is not necessarily a negative experience, it is one that needs sensitive support. Peer support in young carers' groups can be particularly valuable as well as short breaks for the young carer.

SERVICE USERS AS VOLUNTEERS

We will consider the general role of volunteers in social work in the next chapter, but at this point let us note the value that volunteering can bring both to service users and to the people with whom they volunteer. The experiences of service users can be especially useful to other people in similar circumstances and volunteering is a gift of time and experience.

It is a feature of many social work groups that past members are invited to share their experiences ('what a group like this did for me in the past and how I have managed since then') as a way of motivating current group members. The latter learn from a role model who has made a success of their group experience and the volunteer returns the favour of past help.

Of course, it is important that volunteers are not exploited and that the distinction is carefully made between volunteering and working in a role that should be paid. For people who are claiming benefits, the latter could trigger an allegation that the person has 'notional earnings' and could therefore affect their income. Reimbursement of actual expenses, as opposed to a daily allowance which might or might not be spent, will not affect means-tested benefits. As long as they are available for work they are usually able to volunteer and it can be a good way to prepare for formal, paid work.

WHERE DO SOCIAL WORKERS AND CLIENTS MEET?

HOME VISITS

Social workers and service users can meet wherever they choose, but it is most likely to be either in the person's own home or the worker's office. Seeing someone in their own home has many mutual advantages: it is convenient for service users, especially if travel or leaving their home is problematic, and it can feel more comfortable to talk about their situation in familiar surroundings. For the social worker a home visit helps them to see people in context, to understand their situations in a more rounded way and, where appropriate, to see other people in the person's life. Home visits keep workers rooted – in touch with the poverty that many people endure, the communality or nuisance of neighbours, the nearness or distance from amenities such as public transport. All of these are important in social work and they all contribute to the social worker's rounded understanding of a person's situation.

However, there are times when it is beneficial to meet away from a person's home. Social work groups often make use of the neutral space offered by, say, a community centre. Here, there is no host or guest, and all must aim for a common ownership of the space. Social workers know the value, too, of a car ride with a child or young person, sitting side by side to talk about things that might be difficult face to face, and with the sense of privacy that comes in a moving car.

So, the question of where social work happens is not neutral. Where there is a choice it needs to be exercised thoughtfully and with everybody's safety in mind.

ON A CASELOAD

HOW LONG DO YOU HAVE A SOCIAL WORKER FOR?

If you live in one neighbourhood for a length of time you might see the same doctor for many years, even decades. I have had the same dentist since 1976. However, as we explored at the beginning of this chapter, social work is not a universal service and social workers are under considerable pressure to ration their time strictly. The benefits of some short-term methods of intervention have been proven and, of course, it is important to avoid drift; even so, it would be interesting to know the impact of community-based social work practices like general practitioner surgeries, in which local citizens could have access to a social worker merely by residence in a certain area rather than by overcoming eligibility criteria.

Social workers should always remember that, unless they are working in very informal street work or residential care, they usually see service users for a relatively small proportion of that person's week, just a 'snapshot' of their lives; and, because of the push to move people off caseloads quickly, it is hard for social workers to develop long-standing relationships with service users. For all of these reasons, it is important to caution against making life-changing decisions for people after only minimal contact.

ELIGIBILITY AND RATIONING

There are legislative and policy frameworks to help decide who is eligible for social work and who is not, but the decision about where the bar is set (often referred to as a threshold) is generally decided by the availability of resources. Since the 1980s social and economic policy has put more of the UK's increasing wealth into individual pockets than the public purse; so it is paradoxical that as society's wealth has generally increased, the bar for access to social services has been raised rather than lowered. For example, in 2010 it was widely reported that by the following year local councils would be disregarding 'moderate care needs'. In other words, services would be restricted to people who face severe difficulties ('critical or substantial care needs', to use the jargon). What happens in practice in this game is that many people whose needs were assessed as moderate are upgraded to substantial so that they can continue to 'meet eligibility criteria' and, therefore, receive vital social services.

Defining need used to be part of the social work professional role but it has increasingly been taken away from the profession to be governed by procedures. *Fair Access to Care Services* guidance has four categories of need in the UK: critical, substantial, moderate and low. *Critical* is described as 'people are unable to carry out vital personal care tasks; life is or will be threatened; serious abuse or neglect has occurred or will occur'; *low* as 'people are unable to carry out one or two personal care tasks; one or two family or social roles cannot be undertaken'. The social work role is to assess people's needs in line with these categories and on this basis decisions will be taken about what services will be made available, or not. Any remaining discretion largely concerns how social workers can stretch or interpret the criteria on behalf of the service user. It is the social worker who usually breaks the news to people that they are no longer eligible to receive a service.

CASE CLOSED

In the 1970s research indicated that many clients did not know that their cases were 'closed'. This is unlikely to be the case in current times; even so, endings can be difficult, with a confusing array of emotions for service user and social worker. Endings are better if they are planned and some methods of social work practice develop a likely timescale right at the beginning of contact, so that the ending can be seen as something to work towards, planned and anticipated.

Boundaries can be blurred if social workers meet ex-clients in social situations. Of course, it is good for people to catch up with the latest news and developments, but if any new social work seems called for it is important that this is formalised as a new piece of work.

THEMES

DILEMMAS IN SOCIAL WORK

Social workers face dilemmas regularly in their everyday work and these dilemmas are frequently a complex mix of ethics, epistemology and technology; in other words, a judgement about what is the right thing to do, what knowledge there is that bears on the case, and how decisions and judgements can be put into practice.

In every field of social work practice there are dilemmas. Social workers often operate in highly contested areas, where the evidence is scant and contradictory and contextual. Here are some examples:

> What advice does social work have for adoptive parents wishing to change the first name of their adoptive child? Practice wisdom might suggest that this could affect the child's identity adversely, but is there any research to throw light on this hypothesis? Is naming a child part of the bonding process and, if so, is it right to encourage adoptive parents to rename? Would a good outcome be provided by adding an adoptive forename whilst keeping the original first name as a middle name?

> What should a social worker do if they think that the package of care that a service user has arranged puts that service user at risk? The trade-off between a person's right to make their own decisions, even when they entail risks, and the responsibilities of social workers to safeguard people who are vulnerable is a recurring theme in social work theory and practice.

> What does social work have to say about the use of global positioning systems (GPS) to track the movements of people who are confused and experiencing dementia? Does the reassurance that it can provide for the relatives of confused people outweigh concerns about tagging being an infringement of human rights where consent has not been given? Is the stigma of tagging outweighed by the safety? Indeed, is it tagging or is it more a case of 'safer walking' (the term used by the Alzheimer's Society)? Who will pay the costs of the device and who is liable when the technology fails to safeguard an individual?

These kinds of ethical, practical, legal, technological and economic questions are a regular feature of social work, all of which make it such a fascinating profession.

Social workers face dilemmas in terms of the boundaries between their professional and their personal lives. For example, a social worker bumps into an ex-client and learns that the new social worker is doing a very poor job. The quandary lies between wanting to help someone you care about, and not wishing to blur professional boundaries. Turn back to Chapter 1 (page 15) for more examples of morally ambiguous circumstances.

HARD TO REACH OR SELDOM HEARD

Some people are in circumstances that make them 'hard to reach' by formal social work services. Examples are young carers, street people, refugees, travellers (Roma), people diagnosed with personality disorders, and those who do not speak or read the dominant language in a society. All, for various reasons, are unlikely to be aware of the services that might be available or know how to make use of them or want to use them. They might not find them compatible or welcoming.

The term used for these groups, 'hard to reach', can imply that they are making themselves inaccessible, whereas the central problem is often the failure of the services to reach out, to adapt and lose their fortress mentality. For this reason, some prefer to use the term 'seldom heard' for those people who could avail themselves of social work if social work services chose to hear them.

RACE, ETHNICITY AND DIVERSITY

Harassment on grounds of race, ethnic origins, colour or nationality is 'unwanted conduct that has the purpose or effect of violating a person's dignity; or creating an intimidating, hostile, degrading, humiliating or offensive environment for that person'. Social workers have a duty to promote racial equality. Ethnic minorities are, by and large, well represented in social work, comprising 21 per cent of students enrolled on social work degree courses in England in 2009, though they are much less in evidence as senior managers, so there is still much to do to advance equality. In the wider society, ethnic minorities are more likely than the white population to live in poverty, to suffer unemployment and to experience mental ill-health.

The term 'race' is understood to be much more subtly fractured than the monolithic way it is has sometimes been understood. For example, describing people of South Asian descent in the UK as 'black' hid the differences in the circumstances of these groups from, say, African-Caribbean black people; and, further, within the South Asian group itself, the impact of poverty and unemployment falls differentially – less on people of Indian descent and more on Pakistani and Bangladeshi peoples. Most social work practitioners have known differences and commonalities between and within social groups to be highly complex and to transgress boundaries, and this view from the ground is now more widely accepted.

In Chapter 1 (page 29) we considered the social work response in matters of race using a specific example of an 11-year-old boy who had been turned away from his first day at secondary school for wearing his hair in cornrows. The reformist tradition has the social worker working with the family to help them come to terms with the policy, whilst the radical tradition would focus on the school's discriminatory and oppressive policies and perceptions. As so often, social work's task appears practical but is equally philosophical: to redefine social meanings, in this case from one meaning that is understood as a question of fashion to another meaning rooted in race, and to move from a perception of threat to a celebration of diversity.

Social work emphasises respect for different cultural practices, but it is important not to allow unfamiliarity with these practices to inhibit judgement; for instance, if these practices threaten the well-being of a child, such as enforced fasting as deliverance from perceived witchcraft. Behaviours that are attributed in Western terms to, say, autism are often explained quite differently in other cultures. It is important to establish mutual respect, starting with the social worker becoming familiar with the parallel explanations, as the one set of beliefs does not necessarily exclude the other and both may be held at the same time. Social workers must avoid stereotypical assumptions that, for instance, the extended family is automatically helping and supportive 'because in this culture that's what they do'. Social work recognises and understands diversity within the white community, too: 'ethnic' is not a synonym for 'black'.

There is a balance to be struck between consumer choice in social work and the rights of workers, especially black social workers who face discrimination from some service users. The sensitive ethnic matching of social worker to service user is a different matter from capitulating to a racist demand that the worker is not black.

GENDER

Women and feminism have been absolutely central in the development of social work, as explored in Chapter 1. Social work is a largely female profession, both in the numbers of social workers (about 90 per cent in the UK), but also in the nature of the profession. The skills and attributes that a social worker needs (which are sketched in more detail in Chapter 5) are often seen as 'feminine'.

Beyond social work, in the larger society, women provide the bulk of social care, whether informal and unpaid or formal and paid. About 3–4 million carers are women, that is about 58 per cent of the total, and of the estimated 662,000 carers who combine part-time work with caring, 89 per cent are female. One in five people give up paid work in order to provide care and the vast majority of these are women, too. Women's need for social care is also greater, given their greater longevity and higher incidence of mental ill-health.

As with race, so with gender it is important to have an understanding that the categories of 'women' and 'men' are not monolithic. There are many identities within these gender terms; the experience of a working-class white woman is likely to differ from that of a middle-class black woman, and within these subgroups there are further differences and commonalities, right down to personal identities. Oppressive, paternalistic communities are identified as male, and for good reason, but there are many 'masculinities', many expressions of manhood. Men can be feminists and can feel at home in social work without losing a masculine identity.

The absence of men as practitioners and as service users contributes to a perception that men are viewed negatively in social work. I was careful in my own practice to involve and implicate men who were significant to the social work, even if this usually took extra effort, for example working in the evening. Men and social workers can be complicit in avoiding each other, and though the consequences are not easy to compute, it is likely that this results in missed opportunities to strengthen the work and to bring a wide section of the community into the experience of social work and an understanding of what it is.

RISK AND SAFEGUARDING

Notions of risk are central to social work. Whether it is children remaining in their families, people with severe mental health problems staying in their communities or confused, older people in their own homes, there are many finely balanced risks, with sometimes severe consequences if the balance is misjudged. There are also risks, of course, in removing and resettling people into 'safe' environments.

Social workers help people to balance and manage these risks. They do this in a social context, one which has become increasingly averse to risk and where blame is quickly sought and attached, as we saw in the previous chapter. This does not aid cool decision-making and probably increases the number of poor decisions. It has spawned a search for the holy grail of a risk assessment tool or matrix that will somehow take the risk out of risk. Social workers should be judged on the quality of their decision-making, not the outcomes, because the factors that affect the outcomes are just too broad and unknowable – the 'wicked problems' discussed in the first chapter.

The other side to taking risks is the responsibility to provide protection to people who are considered to be vulnerable. This tends to be referred to as 'safeguarding' in UK social work. Risk and safeguarding are not just social work concepts, of course. A stark example was provided recently in the UK when it was suggested that authors (many of them famous names) should be checked with the Criminal Records Bureau before being allowed into schools to talk with children about their writing.

In established and stable communities, people are likely to find protection within their own neighbourhood rather than having to rely on formal systems like the social services. In some cases, an appeal to 'community safeguarding' is seen as a way of broadening awareness and responsibility for looking out for others. The 'Jim's milk has been there a while. Who cares?' campaign is one such example (from the 'I Care' campaign in Barking and Dagenham, east London). This is also a good example of the interplay of social policy and economic policy and the ways in which one can undermine the other; the social role played by doorstep milk deliveries is undercut by economic policies that encourage supermarkets that do not provide these deliveries.

PHYSICAL CONTACT

Physical contact is a significant part of the way we communicate with one another. However, such contact can be construed in different ways and, like any form of communication, professionals must use it sensitively. False accusations against professionals have contributed to a risk-averse culture, with some social work managers instructing staff never to risk any physical contact, especially with children. However, if a social worker hopes to show a child that it is safe for that child to trust the worker, then it should be safe enough for the worker to touch the child. It is a chance to model what is safe touch, so the child might know the difference between safe and unsafe touch. Hugs and arms around shoulders can provide much-needed reassurance and comfort.

RESTRAINT

Most people think of restraint in physical terms, such as the holding of another person in such a way that they cannot move or lash out. However, in social work it covers a wider range of actions. For instance:

> Staff in a residential home use a wheelchair for a resident who is capable of walking to the dining room 'because it's quicker'. In fact, they are restraining her from walking, as walking is an activity she can do and enjoys. The first step with restraint is, therefore, to recognise it.

Emergency situations can require the use of immediate restraint, but those situations that develop over some time are the most challenging to decide whether restraint is justified and, if so, what kind. The first principle is that people exercise choice; considerations about restraint are necessary when there is doubt about the mental capacity of the person to make these judgements and the risks that this might pose for themselves and others. It is important first to search for options other than restraint.

VIOLENCE

In the UK, when the police are called to an incident of domestic violence where there are children present, they must notify social services. However, only five per cent of all such police notifications result in social work interventions (NSPCC study, UK, 2010). Social work has a role to play in work with the people who commit violence (the perpetrators) but there is often reluctance on the part of a mainly female workforce to undertake this and a reliance on specialist domestic violence support services where these exist.

As well as working with people who commit violent acts within their families, social workers sometimes experience violence themselves; one in five of all UK workers who are 'signed off' (unable to attend work) because of work-related assaults is employed in social care. These figures do not include verbal assaults and incidents where workers were struck without major injury, as this information is not collected in any national database.

SEX

One of the many controversial topics in social work is sex. Here is an example of the controversy:

> Should it be possible for the individual budgets that we discussed earlier in the chapter (personalisation) to be spent on sexual relations? Social work aims to empower people, so if a disabled person wishes to seek sexual fulfillment, should social work assist this by helping to arrange a sex worker?

It is a complex issue in which social work values about possible exploitation, the rights of individuals to equal access to services, and the law (upholding human rights as opposed to the legality of arranging sexual services) all have a bearing. The case of a young man with learning disabilities who wanted to use part of his income support to fund a sex trip to Amsterdam was posted on an online site in 2010 and prompted strong debate (http:/bit.ly/bR9v8r).

Sex between a social worker and a service user is more straightforward, in that it is hard to think of any circumstances when this would be acceptable. Whilst service users should not be patronised as incapable of making their own decisions, the particular contract of trust between a professional and the person with whom they are working rules out the crossing of this line. The relative power of the social worker means that sex (and, indeed, love) in the professional–service user relationship cannot be construed in the same way as it would be outside this relationship. However, a sexual relationship between a social worker and an ex-client starts to enter a grey area in which one could construct circumstances when this could be OK.

A third area of controversy can be found in the sexual behaviour of social workers outside their work:

Should a social worker be barred from the profession, temporarily or permanently, if they employ a sex worker?

In 2010 a UK social worker was struck off the social care register (i.e. prevented from practising as a social worker) because he had been caught engaging in sexual activity with a sex worker. However, he was already being investigated following accusations of inappropriate conduct involving a female service user.

WHAT DO SERVICE USERS WANT FROM SOCIAL WORK?

Some key messages have emerged from studies of service users' views of social work and what they want from it. Almost universally, they want the human face of social work and they criticise bureaucratic and defensive social work, where social workers 'have to speak to my manager' before any decision can be taken. This comment from a man who was in care as a youth is typical:

'My social worker ... started working with me when I was eight and when she finally moved on she insisted we remain in touch. Our relationship would be frowned upon today; she would be accused of blurring the professional line. But it was this relationship that saved me.'

(the *Guardian*, 10/8/10: 23)

Service users want their social workers to be reliable, punctual, approachable and they want them to stay around long enough to develop a relationship. Although it is not always stated in these explicit terms, it seems that they appreciate a social worker who can be assertive with their own agency and fight their corner when it comes to securing resources. They want honesty. Even when the social worker is making decisions with which parents disagree (for example, to remove the child from the home), one of the most important factors for parents is the way social workers conduct themselves. They appreciate honest, direct communications, even if they disagree with the message.

Social workers need to understand how difficult it can be for service users to participate freely in meetings that are packed with professionals. A man who is caring for his elderly father notes:

'Meetings with professionals are tough ... You feel like a bad lad at school in front of a board of school governors.'

(Community Care, 9/9/10: 22)

In meetings where there are many different professions represented, social workers should be particularly well placed to help professionals and service users to communicate with one another.

Service users have had a uniquely central place in the social work profession, the first to involve service users in a systematic way in the education and training of its professionals. However, the pressures on social workers to retreat into the supposed safety of procedure and formula endangers what is essential to social work – the humanity that is experienced when social work is free to express itself creatively.

IN CONCLUSION

This chapter surveyed the wide range of circumstances that can bring somebody into the world of social work. We explored the controversy about the terms used to describe the people who use social work services and the ambivalent, sometime hostile, feelings that people have towards social work. The complexities of gender, race and ethnicity were explored in relation to social work. The chapter has considered some examples of social work dilemmas: making judgements about the right thing to do, finding the relevant knowledge, and knowing how decisions can best be put into practice, particularly when risks are taken. Finally, we described what research and experience suggests people want from their contacts with social work.

FURTHER READING

R. Adams, L. Dominelli and M. Payne (eds), *Social Work: Themes, Issues and Critical Debates* (3rd edition), New York: Palgrave, 2009.

A good introduction to some of the major debates in current social work theory and practice.

W. Devore and E.G. Schlesinger, *Ethnic-Sensitive Social Work Practice* (4th edition), Boston: Allyn and Bacon, 1999.
This American book remains a classic text and explores ethnic and class factors in social work practice.

M. Doel and L. Best, *Experiencing Social Work: Learning From Service Users*, London: Sage, 2008.
Tells the stories of a variety of service users who have had positive experiences of social work, and the lessons to be learned from these accounts.

J.E. Mayer and N. Timms, *The Client Speaks*, London: Routledge and Kegan Paul, 1970.
A seminal work that exposed the different ways in which social workers and their clients viewed their work; it is still a powerful read.

G. Ruch, D. Turney and A. Ward (eds), *Relationship-Based Social Work*, London: Jessica Kingsley, 2010.
An edited book that affirms the central place of 'relationship' in social work practice, using examples from many of the service user groups presented earlier in this chapter.

S.M. Shardlow and P. Nelson (eds), *Introducing Social Work*, Poole: Russell House Publishing, 2005.
A concise introduction to specific settings in which social work is practised. The book includes chapters on children and families, community care for older people, probation work, mental health and disability.

SOME RELATED WEBLINKS

www.dh.gov.uk/health/category/policy-areas/social-care and *www.education.gov.uk/publications/standard/Childrenandfamilies/Page1* Publications about social work can be downloaded from the Department of Health and the Department for Education websites.

www.stayingput.uk.net The 'Staying Put' scheme.

www.scie.org.uk The Social Care Institute for Excellence (Scie) provides research briefings and good practice guidelines concerning specific service user groups.

www.shapingourlives.org.uk Shaping Our Lives is a UK network of service users and disabled people.

REFERENCES

Akinsanya, D. 'Social Work needs a Human Face', the *Guardian*, 10/8/10: 23.

Community Care (2010), 'Poll results: is the new NSPCC chief executive right to admit that we may never end child cruelty', 25/2/10: 14.

The Guardian (2010), 'Foster carer's diary – August', 27/11/10: 23.

Guardian Weekend (2010), 'Foster carer's diary – July', 27/11/10: 23.

Pitt, V. 'A conflict of best interests', *Community Care*, 9/9/10: 22.

4

A PROFESSION OR A CAREER; A CALLING OR A JOB

WHAT SOCIAL WORKERS DO AND HOW SOCIAL WORK IS ORGANISED

This chapter presents the many facets of social work. It explains social work practice, the daily experience of social workers and the practical organisation and management of social work services (which will be referred to as social services) and how social work is regulated.

A PROFESSION

WHAT IS A PROFESSION?

One of the defining characteristics of a profession is the degree of autonomy experienced by the individual practitioners. To what extent can they organise their own day and take decisions using their own judgement? Another characteristic of a profession is the monopoly it holds over a particular area of knowledge. This is usually a complex mix of theoretical knowledge applied in practice. Neurosurgeons have highly specialised knowledge of the workings of the human nervous system and they are able to intervene (in brain surgery) to put this knowledge to practical use. In one sense, plumbers have the same mix of knowledge and practical skill but plumbing is not considered to be a profession.

Perhaps the key to successfully claiming professional status is the ability to persuade others that it is earned, in other words an occupational group's capacity to exert power. A neurosurgeon may be no better at plumbing than a plumber is at neurosurgery, but the former earns a good deal more money, is more difficult to replace and demands high grades to enter a lengthy period of training. This gives the neurosurgeon more power than the plumber.

Alternatively, perhaps it is more a question of the ability to gain the trust of the wider community in your desire to act in the broader interest rather than your own. This is regarded as professional integrity and it is demonstrated by, amongst other things, the existence of a professional ethical code.

Where does social work stand as a profession? The increase in the use of procedures to govern the way social workers perform their tasks is seen as compromising their autonomy and possibly as evidence that social work is not a full profession, but a para-profession. Yet doctors are also increasingly subject to governance from outside their profession without a loss of professional status.

Social work has long experienced doubts about its knowledge and theory base. It is reassuring to perform something seemingly clear-cut like neuroscience (or, indeed, plumbing), where the set of skills is most definitely defined and observable. Social work borrows from so many different disciplines, as we saw in Chapter 1, falling short of occupying any single specific territory.

Does social work earn the respect due to a profession? The pay of social workers is nothing special, though – like neurosurgeons and unlike plumbers – they are generally in regular employment. Social work has long had a presence in universities and the training is generally at degree level, though in Germany it is excluded from full universities at the higher levels. Social work has an international presence and a growing body of research. There are professional organisations in many countries around the world and also an international association. Despite legitimate concerns, on balance social work can be considered to be a profession.

PROFESSIONALISM

Members of a profession are expected to show professionalism in their conduct. This is usually taken to include upholding the profession's reputation, managing the boundaries between the personal and the professional and keeping professional knowledge up to date. Professionalism is the first of nine core standards for social workers set out by the Social Work Reform Board in England in 2010.

There is a view that the notion of professionalism is elitist and results in the distancing of social workers from the people they work with. This is perhaps most strongly held by those who see social work as a calling. However, professionalism need not mean clinical distance; social work ranges widely between roles – from advocate to investigator, for instance – whilst remaining sensitive, approachable and authoritative. The dossier of a winner of the Social Worker of the Year award (UK) included a testimonial from a girl on a care order living in the same street as the social worker who escaped her home life by popping round to the home of the social worker several times a week for dinner. Professionalism does not have to mean distance.

It is not possible to be fully professional in a workplace which does not share the profession's values, so responsibility is shared with the professional's employer. I had to resign from my first job as a qualified social worker because of the lack of professionalism of the organisation where I worked. The clients could be protected from some of the worst effects of the organisation; nevertheless, accepting a pay cheque from an organisation is tantamount to lending it your support and the time can come when it is no longer right to do so. Professionalism means having first loyalty to the profession's values, which in themselves hold the community's interests paramount over personal interests or those of any employing organisation.

DRESS CODE

Dress is a challenge for social workers because they can easily find themselves in court, in a service user's home, and leading a street-based activity group all in the same day, with widely different dress needs. In a poll asking respondents to choose whether smart shoes or trainers were the most appropriate attire for social workers, smart shoes came out top (76 per cent); nevertheless, a sizeable minority (24 per cent) opted for trainers ('Dress for success', *Community Care*, 9/12/10: 28).

The social work profession does not have a dress code. An instruction from one English local authority to 'carefully consider their work attire' and dress more conservatively is, therefore, a rare example of the issue being openly addressed.

We might like to think that appearance is secondary and that what is on the inside really counts; however, most of the world makes its assessment by what it sees and a chunk of that comes from what is worn. This was brought home to me when I was told that I had to wear a tie even though my work involved me with adolescents in the downtown area of a large American city in hot, sticky conditions. The agency in which I experienced unprofessional practice insisted on conventional professional attire, so the one is not a guarantee of the other.

A CAREER OR A CALLING

I was not certain that I wanted to be a social worker until I was employed as an unqualified social worker for a year in a rural English county. I cannot, therefore, say that I had a 'calling', but nor did I have a strong sense of career. I knew I wanted to work with people (often disparaged as naive when stated by would-be students at interview, but I always have a sympathy with them), but no strong sense of how that might take shape. I suspect that not many people choose social work purely on the basis of career as there are better-paid, less stressful ones to choose from.

CAREER STRUCTURE

A career structure is important for the survival of any profession, whatever the motivations of people seeking to join. An opportunity for progression helps to retain them in the profession. The notion of 'levels' was first established in the UK following a series of public sector strikes in 1978–79, with newly qualified social workers starting at level one and able to progress to level three. However, the notion of senior practitioner has been underdeveloped in social work and there is no equivalent of the consultant in medicine.

The only opportunities for social workers to advance beyond what in most countries is a modest income (though they are very well paid in Ireland, for instance) is to move into senior management or senior academic positions. However, as social work has become less of a state monopoly, new opportunities have been opening for entrepreneurial social workers; for example, providing residential care for older people or specialist treatment centres for children and young people.

TRAINEES, SUPPORT WORKERS AND VOLUNTEERS

My own entry into social work came via paid work as an unqualified worker. These positions often led to trainee positions, in which local authorities in the UK would sponsor promising workers to take up training, either on a full-time or part-time basis, with a commitment to return to the sponsoring authority, usually for two years. This approach has been rediscovered, coined now as 'grow your own', especially in areas with dangerous shortages of social workers, as in some London boroughs.

When I first started as a qualified social worker each team had positions for two social work assistants. More recently, similar posts are likely to be called support workers and this is a good way to test the social work waters; indeed, the fear is that qualified social workers have diminishing contact with actual people and spend more of their time in co-ordinating roles, overseeing 'packages of care', with support workers doing the bulk of the personal work. However, there is a strong reaction in the profession against this trend and in favour of relationship-based work. Accountability for delegated work still lies with the social worker who, therefore, needs to have confidence in the support worker.

Can anyone 'do social work'? Yes and no. In some respects social work is no different from teaching and nursing, as we discussed in Chapter 1, in that parents can teach their children and partners can nurse each other without holding professional qualifications in teaching or nursing. Similarly, volunteers can do social work (it is interesting that there is no verb 'to social work', unlike 'to teach' and 'to nurse'). Volunteers cannot be expected to work with the same complexities as professional social workers but, often, they can bring something that social workers cannot, such as direct experience of the lives of the people with whom they volunteer.

One of the greatest concerns is that volunteers will be exploited as cut-price workers and that they will be asked to do work that is beyond their capabilities. One of my roles as a community-based social worker was to recruit and support a group of volunteers; a very rewarding experience for the volunteers, for the people they volunteered with and for me. It is crucial that volunteers have a specific role, that they are supported, that they meet together regularly for peer support and that they know when to ask for professional social work involvement. It is important to find out what motivates a particular volunteer as this varies from person to person.

As noted in the previous chapter, people receiving state benefits need to check whether volunteering will affect their allowances.

A JOB

Whether social work is a profession or a semi-profession, a calling or a career, it is certainly a job. Indeed, since it became embedded in the apparatus of state welfare, concerns have regularly been expressed that it is being *defined* by its employment. As we shall see in the next chapter, employers in the UK have a strong role in the education of social workers and, therefore, in the shape of social work itself.

THE WORKFORCE

There were over 84,300 social workers registered in England in 2011, about one for every 600 inhabitants; 10,552 in Scotland (one for 490); 5,672 in Wales (one for 530); and 5,323 in Northern Ireland (one for 336). Note that 'registered and qualified' does not necessarily mean practising. In the US social workers held about 642,000 jobs in 2008, one social work job for approximately every 500 inhabitants (United States Bureau of Labor Statistics); about 54 per cent were in healthcare and social assistance industries, and 31 per cent were employed by government agencies. Employment by type of social worker in the US in 2008 was:

Child, family and school social workers   292,600
Medical and public health social workers   138,700
Mental health and substance abuse social workers   137,300
Social workers (all other)   73,400

The 'typical' social worker in the UK in 2011 is a woman in her forties with children, just as it was when the Barclay Committee reported on social work in 1982. This contrasts with the typical media image of a newly qualified graduate with little life experience. In fact, the threat to social work comes, if threat there is, from the demography of its workforce: in Britain fewer than five per cent are younger than 25 and many are in their fifties, and there are few men in social work frontline jobs (see previous chapter), significantly fewer than when I qualified in the 1970s.

RECRUITMENT AND RETENTION

Turnover of social work staff, the 'churn rate', is high at about 15 per cent in the UK, and vacancy rates are generally over 10 per cent. However, they vary considerably from area to area: 4 per cent in Northern Ireland to over 15 per cent in East England; and between different services, with 3 per cent for adult services in Wales and 16.5 per cent for children's services in the West Midlands, though the highest single regional rate was almost 31 per cent for adult services in East England (all 2010 figures). Rates can move quickly over a relatively short period; for instance, down from 14 per cent in Wales in 2005 to 7 per cent in Wales in 2010. Of course, these problems are not unique to social work, with teaching and nursing experiencing similar challenges to recruit and keep their staff.

Once recruited, agencies must find ways to retain their staff to limit turnover. There are obvious advantages to a stable workforce, such as continuity for the service users and the chance to build local knowledge and networks. However, some turnover is also beneficial to introduce new ideas and working practices. It is interesting to speculate what the 'goldilocks' turnover rate might be, i.e. not too little, not too much.

Research suggests that one of the most effective ways for agencies to improve recruitment is to pay attention to the quality of the placements they offer students. The students of today are likely to become the employees of tomorrow if they like what they see. Moreover, staff who are supported in their work as practice educators (teachers of social work on placements) will gain satisfaction from their job and, one can infer, are more likely to stay in it.

EMPLOYMENT AND WORKING CONDITIONS

Research in the UK indicated that social workers had long working hours, excessive workloads and too much bureaucracy. This became the platform for a campaign called the Social Work Contract, an alliance between Unison (the major union for social workers in the

UK) and *Community Care*, a social care magazine. The main demands reflect what can be considered to be acceptable working conditions:

- a manageable caseload;
- guaranteed professional supervision;
- compensation for excess hours worked;
- a right to assistance with professional development;
- decent IT and administrative backup;
- safe working practices;
- support when dealing with stress and traumatic cases.

Time away from the day-to-day work is necessary for social workers to reflect on their work, but they rarely have the contractual right to 10 per cent of their working time, as teachers do, for planning and preparation.

A survey of UK social workers in 2010 found 71 per cent were very or fairly satisfied and 28 per cent were not very or not at all satisfied (*Community Care*, 9/12/10: 4–5). This is perhaps a surprisingly high percentage of reasonably satisfied workers given the fact that the same survey revealed that nearly a quarter of social workers were working more than 45 hours a week, though contracted typically for 35 hours.

AGENCY SOCIAL WORKERS (LOCUMS)

Teams need stability to be effective and it is difficult to reconcile this with the widespread practice in the UK of employing temporary social workers from independent agencies, usually referred to as agency social workers or locums. About 10 per cent of all social work posts in UK local authorities were filled by agency social workers in 2011.

Although locums provide social work agencies with flexibility (they can be bought in and laid off according to fluctuating demand), they are expensive: an estimated £14,400 ($23,000) more than a permanent staff member, which totals between £70m and £140m for the UK. One English county council alone spent an additional £1.5 million in 2010 to recruit two teams of agency social workers to meet an unprecedented increase in referrals to its child protection service.

Locum work gives agency social workers a degree of freedom, but they can also find that they get dumped with the work that no-one else wants to do and that they are short-changed in terms of training and professional development. Whether they are resented or welcomed as an extra pair of hands will probably depend on the extent to which the employer is relying on them: if it is less than 10 per cent they might be welcomed, but over 20 per cent becomes unstable and disrupts continuity for service users.

PAY AND PENSION

The average pay for a UK social worker in 2010 was £33,440 per year ($53,500), with an average of nineteen years' experience (as revealed in the survey cited earlier). The average salary for UK social workers across their lives is £30,040 per year (for nurses it is £29,494, for teachers £36,837 and for doctors £84,451). Results from the 2010 UK Annual Survey of Hours and Earnings show that median annual pay for full-time employees was £25,948. The UK Office of National Statistics reveal no gender gap in social work pay – indeed, women in social work are more likely to be paid 1.4 per cent more than men. This contrasts with 90 per cent of all job types where men's pay is greater than women's for the same work.

In local government in the UK, job roles are allocated points and salaries and graded accordingly. This leaves little scope for local flexibility, so the relatively low basic pay is sometimes supplemented with add-on perks ('market forces supplements'), such as gym membership, childcare vouchers, cycling schemes, golden hellos, retention bonuses and, for some foreign social workers, a free flight home each year. These benefits are not consolidated into the salary, so they can be removed easily if cuts have to be made. However, 77 per cent of public sector employers do not offer these kinds of incentive, so they are not (yet) widespread.

In countries where there are large differences in costs of living from one region to another, public sector salaries are inadequate in the high-cost areas. The UK Labour government introduced a scheme to provide housing for public sector staff, in which nurses had 3,992 loans, teachers 2,817 and the police 892. Social workers competed with fire fighters and transport workers for 311 loans. Whereas teachers were receiving 'golden hellos' of £4,000 in subjects where shortages were experienced, social work enjoyed no such benefits.

The pay of senior managements in social work can be substantial, with directors of social services agencies paid around £120,000 per year. Social workers who work in the public sector in the UK benefit from the local government pension scheme. A percentage of final salary is paid (each year of service counts as one sixtieth of the final salary), though proposals by the 2010 Coalition government to change public sector pensions are meeting concerted opposition.

UNIONS AND INDUSTRIAL RELATIONS

The main public sector union to represent social workers in the UK is Unison (successor to NALGO), which represents 40,000 social workers.

Industrial relations in the public sector in the UK were at their most conflicted in the late 1970s when social workers in selected local authorities voted to strike. Given the vulnerabilities of service users, striking was a difficult decision. Since that period union membership has declined and, along with it, worker power. Even so, in 2010, a scheme to establish an independent social work practice in the English West Midlands was defeated by union opposition, concerned about privatisation and job losses.

A 2010 poll of UK social care workers (a wider workforce than social workers, explained later in this chapter) revealed that 70 per cent of respondents would strike to protect social care. A further poll in 2011 had 46 per cent saying they would support industrial action to oppose a 5 per cent pay cut, with 38 per cent stating they would look for new jobs, and 17 per cent that they would 'grin and bear it' (a poll in *Community Care*, 3/3/11: 13).

HEALTH AND SAFETY

Health and safety has become a bogey in some sections of the press, rather like 'political correctness' (see page 59). It is important, then, to stress that since the Health and Safety at Work Act, 1974, deaths and serious injuries at work have fallen significantly to the extent that the UK enjoys one of the lowest fatal injury rates in Europe.

Since social workers can be exposed to dangerous situations it is important that their safety is paramount. However, the operation of health and safety can be clunky and overly bureaucratic, and documentation for a small risk can be as onerous as for a large one. It needs to be proportionate; if health and safety becomes an unthinking obstacle to innovation then it acquires a bad name.

Sickness has a big impact in a small team and employers need to consider how the health of their social workers can best be protected. Although the total number of people on long-term sick leave is small, one survey found that it accounted for 40 per cent of days lost – and, contrary to general opinion, these long-term absences were not due to stress but to recovery from surgery and long-term treatments for ailments such as cancer.

As a predominantly female profession, there is a particular need for employers of social workers to consider how work can fit around caring responsibilities.

THEMES

ACCOUNTABILITY

The notion of accountability is complex. The first obvious question is, to whom are social workers accountable: the service users; the profession; the employer; themselves; the wider public? The answer is all of these, but the balance between them is fluid and, of course, has a bearing on the earlier questions about whether social work is more a profession or a job. In multi-professional settings, where the social worker's manager might not be a social worker, the issues become more complicated.

Just as important as the direction of accountability is how it is exercised. If a service user has a complaint, should this be addressed to the worker's employer or their professional association? And if a social worker chooses to 'whistleblow' about unprofessional practices in the workplace, how and where should this be done? We will explore issues of professional conduct later.

When social workers are largely employed in the public sector, accountability is closely tied to a notion of *democratic* accountability, since their ultimate employers are elected by local communities. There has been considerable growth in private consultancies, with an increasingly strong grip on inspection and review of social care in the UK (one consultancy had a turnover of £238m in 2009); but with no lines of accountability to democratically elected bodies this raises serious yet infrequently asked questions about the democratic accountability of profit-making organisations in the field of social work.

AUTONOMY

In the professional context, autonomy is interpreted as the capacity to make uncoerced decisions and, with that, the acceptance of responsibility for these decisions. At a broader level it is linked to self-determination, which can refer to a national as well as an individual condition. Social workers are expected to respect the autonomy of service users and, where they are struggling with this, to help them towards self-determination.

These are high ideals and, in practice, severely constrained. Social workers' autonomy is limited by the rise of proceduralism described later, in which the way decisions are made is prescribed and highly formalised – more like painting by numbers than expressive high art. Service users' autonomy is frequently compromised by social workers' concerns about their well-being or the well-being of those around them. This is a kind of social beneficence, in which social workers must judge the balance between their own prescriptions for the well-being of service users against the service user's own choices.

Autonomy is a necessity for social workers in remote locations such as the Scottish islands where 'nipping back to the office' is not an option. There is some evidence that autonomy makes economic sense, too. In a unit where the staff determined their own rota there was a lower rate of absence (sickness etc.) than in similar units where rotas were fixed or issued by the managers.

AUTHORITY

A number of factors conspire to inhibit the exercise of professional authority. One is the general retreat from deferential attitudes as part of the broadening of access to professional education and another is the increased emphasis on the expertise of service users themselves.

These are positive developments and they should not, in themselves, prevent the *appropriate* use of professional authority by social workers. It means that authority must be exercised with more care and subtlety than has sometimes been the case.

Power accrues to the role of the social worker, some of it embedded in the law as we shall see in the next chapter. The challenge for social workers is to recognise their power and to exercise it in ways that provide support and protection yet avoid oppressive practices. Serious Case Reviews, which are held to understand what happened in situations such as child deaths, frequently provide evidence of what can happen when social workers are not capable of exercising authority. Indeed, in the case of Peter Connolly in London in 2009 'the need for authoritative child protection practice' was stated as the first lesson to be learned, with 'authority' repeated in five of the fifteen recommendations.

BUREAUCRACY AND DISCRETION

Protocols and procedures are necessary to ensure that resources are distributed fairly and that a person's experience of a service is not based on the whim or prejudice of the practitioner. Standardisation avoids a 'postcode lottery', when the quality of services differs from area to area. However, a professional service must also take account of people's varying needs, and social workers must be able to exercise discretion in order to respond to these variations.

There is a growing consensus that the balance between bureaucracy and discretion is wrong. A major review of social work in the UK in 2010 (the Munro review) highlighted bureaucracy as stifling social workers' ability to be professional. The regime of targets, centralised policymaking and regular diktats reacting to the latest moral panic has lengthened the lists of bullet-points that prescribe practice. For some social workers the experience is less that of a professional exercising judgement and more a civil servant administering a set of procedures. However, fears have been expressed that some social workers have lost their professional confidence and hide behind the paperwork as an excuse not to have to engage in face-to-face work.

Here is an illustration of the clash between professionalism and proceduralism:

It is accepted wisdom that speaking with someone on their own can expose concerns about possible abuse that would not surface if the interview were conducted with the person's carer present, as this person might be the source of that abuse. A London council now includes 'Lone Appointments' as part of its 'Standard operating procedures for social workers', developed by the 'Safeguarding Team'.

Probably 99 out of 100 social workers know this practice wisdom and use it: what we do not know is whether having a 'Lone Appointments' procedure actually affects the work of the reprobate one in 100; more critically, we do not know the impact of yet another procedure on the morale of the other 99 who are already complying.

The lessons from the illustration of the Lone Appointment procedure are complex. At a philosophical level, is it better to know the practice or to know the procedure? There are different kinds of 'know'. I know that I like plums, and I know the capital of Ecuador, but I have to *recall* the latter. The process of recalling a prescribed procedure (one amongst dozens, possibly hundreds of other procedures) is quite different from *knowing* what is good practice. The procedure, designed to catch the failing one in 100, might in fact fail to do so. (Of course, we cannot know the actual percentage of social workers who need this kind of procedural prescription and those who formulated the Lone Appointments procedure might claim that it is much higher than one in 100. However, we do know that contact with situations that go wrong leads to 'perception bias', a tendency to think that this represents general practice.) Additionally, this procedure does not provide a protocol for those one in 100 occasions when it is *right* to interview the person in the presence of their carer. The reasons why this might be the case are so subtle, complex and specific to the situation that it is not possible to provide a meaningful procedure for it.

The example above illustrates a growing tendency for good practice to be defined by people in specialist or management positions. A reaction to the deluge of prescription from central government and regulatory bodies is often not to create more frontline workers to work with the problem but to create more specialist managers to *manage* the problem, especially to manage the way the problem looks as though it is being dealt with.

'Bureaucracy' is often used as shorthand for rules and regulations we do not like. For instance:

> In 2010 the UK Coalition government called for a war on 'foster carer red tape', complaining about the restrictions imposed on foster carers by some councils and aiming to reduce the size of adoption and fostering panels. Clearly, requiring foster carers to seek permission each time they want to take their child for a haircut is unnecessarily controlling, but there are also good reasons why foster care should be strictly regulated.

Although the restriction on professional discretion is one of the biggest challenges to social work, we should take care that attacks on bureaucracy are discerning.

TEAMWORK

Most social workers are not independent clinicians. They usually work in teams and these teams are increasingly likely to consist of members from other professions.

Teams differ in the ways they work, influenced by the team culture and the team leader. Being organised in a team does not automatically lead to *teamwork*:

> I witnessed two teams who worked in neighbouring districts with similar demographics: one team had an individualistic approach in which each did his or her own thing; the other met at the beginning of each working day to look through the previous day's 'referrals' (people referred for a social work service) to decide how to respond and to plan the working day, sometimes including joint visits where two social workers work together. It was a good advert for teamwork, as the latter team never had any referrals waiting, whilst the former had a depressingly high stack of unallocated cases.

Working as a team can provide better continuity for service users as well as a quicker response.

Team leaders face difficult choices about how to use the various team members: do you always give the most competent member the most complex cases or do you make sure others in the team have an opportunity to learn and to grow? Making space for team members to reflect on their work and to review their priorities on a regular basis helps the team as a whole to grow. The team's importance is being recognised once again in the UK, where an annual 'health check' for teams is recommended by the Social Work Reform Board.

WORKLOAD

The quantity of work that a social worker has on their plate is often referred to as their workload, and the number of cases (individual pieces of work) as their caseload. It is problematic to measure workload and although the size of a caseload is an indicator of this load, it is unreliable, as one case is often not equal to another in complexity and the time it consumes. 16 per cent of social workers in a UK poll in 2010 claimed they had caseloads numbering above forty and 90 per cent reported that high caseloads were affecting their ability to practise good social work (*Community Care*, 9/9/10: 5). The same case can vary in the course of a week from low demand to high stress. How many individual cases is equivalent to leading a group?

Workload management systems have found waves of popularity since the 1970s, especially amongst social work managers who see them as, at best, a way to distribute work equitably and, at worst, a way to expose poor and inefficient workers. However, completing the documentation for the workload recording system can be complex, so that it actually adds to the workload; and, as it usually depends on self-report, it is open to misrepresentation, deliberate or otherwise.

It is not in any way similar to measuring the numbers of loaves a worker can clear off a conveyor belt in a given time, so it is tempting for social workers to stop trying to quantify workload. However, the knowledge is important. Regular supervision, frequent team discussion of the team's work and a collaborative allocation system of new work are much more likely to increase awareness of the distribution of workloads across the team and to develop a consensus about fair balance and reasonable caseload size. This can nurture transparency about workloads that is qualitatively meaningful rather than falsely numerical. Teamworking is likely to give individual social workers more confidence to speak up when they feel pressured and to know when it is right to say no to more work.

MANAGEMENT AND LEADERSHIP

Formerly, social workers were generally managed by qualified social workers. Certainly, in the UK at the time of the large public agencies known as social services departments, team managers were always qualified social workers, as were virtually all senior managers. There was a legal requirement that the director of social services was a qualified social worker.

As social work services have moved strongly into specialisms, social workers are increasingly finding themselves managed by someone from outside the profession, though they should always seek *supervision* from a qualified social worker. Conversely, there are also opportunities for a social worker to become the manager of, say, a district hospital (as has happened in Wales). There is much controversy about whether it matters that social workers are managed by their own profession. On the one hand, the kinds of skills that social workers bring to their work are useful ones to lead teams; on the other hand, the skills of managing are often seen as transferable from one service area to another and management is viewed as its own profession. Managerial and professional responsibilities should be separated, so professional supervision is given by social workers.

Social workers do not necessarily have managerial skills and they need further education and training to make this transition successfully. (Post-qualifying education is considered in the next chapter.) At the level of team leader, qualified social workers are most likely to understand the pressures of frontline work and to be able to 'hold' (emotionally as well as practically) unallocated cases. As qualified social workers, they can provide good role models for the social work team members. At senior management levels, the ability to secure resources, to strategise and to provide leadership are more important and not necessarily part of a qualified social worker's range.

Managers who respect the professionalism of their staff and avoid the worst excesses of managerialism are likely to be valued by their social workers. Good leadership comes from being able to see beyond your own agency and to communicate realistic strategies that inspire others, too.

A 'glass ceiling' for black and ethnic minority staff has been identified in terms of moving into management jobs. For example, only four out of 152 adult services directors in England in 2011 were from a black and ethnic minority group – that is 2.6 per cent, compared to 17 per cent of all registered social workers and 22 per cent of care workers. People from black and ethnic minorities make up 12 per cent of the general population in England.

SOCIAL WORK PRACTICE

How do social workers work? You probably have a reasonably good idea how teachers teach and how doctors take a history to arrive at a diagnosis, but what do social workers actually do when they meet with their service users? What does social work practice look like?

It is a simple question with numerous answers. Let us consider our response first by investigating the dominant perspective in social work, then the notion of social work methods and the environments or milieux in which social work occurs.

STRENGTHS PERSPECTIVE

The pre-eminent approach in social work is known as the strengths perspective. What this means in practice is that social workers aim to work with people to identify their strengths and to work with these. In past times the tendency was to focus on the psychopathy of people's situations, i.e. what was 'wrong' with them, and to emphasise problems and dysfunction. This was summed up in the term 'problem families'.

Despite the difficulties that bring people to the attention of social work, there is recognition that often they have exhibited enormous resilience. A person raising children on their own in a tower block with very little income has often demonstrated greater self-sufficiency than, say, the social worker who has come to help. Working with strengths to achieve solutions (rather than ferreting out deficits to identify problems) does not mean that social workers ignore the difficulties and the hurdles, but that they start with the person's competences and work from there.

The strengths perspective also views people's current difficulties through the prism of critical social policy, that is, an understanding of the social structures that exclude certain groups from the main-stream. In this way, the personal is seen as part of the social; individual troubles related to public ills. In recent times there has been a resurgence of the notion of the relationship as central to social work (known as 'building rapport'), not as an end in itself but as the key to unlocking the service user's strengths.

SOCIAL WORK METHODS

What empirical evidence we have about what actually happens in service users' encounters with social work suggests that workers do not make regular use of systematic methods and that prescribed agency procedures predominate. This has diminished opportunities for practitioners to use methodologies derived from social work practice.

There are very few methods that have been 'home-grown' from within social work. Most have been borrowed and adapted from other disciplines, such as cognitive behavioural treatment (CBT) from psychology or solution-focused practice from counselling. The main disciplines that have contributed to social work methods are sociology, psychology, education and systems theories. As we have noted, much social work practice emphasises the development and use of the relationship between the social worker and the service user.

One of the home-grown methods is called task-centred social work, a member of the problem-solving family of methods:

> The problems that bring the service user and the social worker together are carefully explored. Together, the worker and service user agree goals that the service user wants to achieve and that are realisable, along with an agreed time limit by which the goals can realistically be achieved. All of this (the details of the problems and the attendant goals) is usually written down in a contract or agreement. At each session a series of tasks are agreed that will help to achieve the agreed goals and, there-fore, reduce the identified problems. The social worker, the service user and sometimes other significant people in the person's life agree to undertake tasks. Progress on the tasks is reviewed at each subsequent session. The theory underpinning task-centred practice derives from learning theories and the value base is one of a partnership, empower-ment and a strong working relationship. The method has been exten-sively researched and it has been evaluated positively in very different circumstances.

English is an imprecise language and 'method' is especially slippery. For instance, 'early intervention' is often incorrectly described as a method, whereas it is a general strategy or approach, in which many different kinds of method might be used. Tools are often described as methods, such as 'Distance Travelled': this is 'a method' of measuring progress, but is strictly speaking a tool, used as part of a broader, systematic method.

> Family Group Conferencing is a method that has been adapted by western social work from Maori practices in New Zealand. It recognises the significance of the wider family in a child's life and the fact that the more workable and sustainable solutions to problems in the care of a child are more likely to arise from the child's wider kin. The professional's work is to bring the wider family together and to provide the circumstances whereby the child's extended family can arrive at a decision about the best care for the child. This can be challenging for some professionals' understanding of their role.

MILIEU: INDIVIDUAL, FAMILY, GROUP, COMMUNITY

The classic pillars of social work are casework, family work, groupwork and community work. These are self-evident in terms of the environments in which they occur and they were what a social worker from the 1960s would have understood as specialisms. Although statistics are hard to come by, the majority of social workers in Western countries work at the level of the individual and, in the US, social work practice has become very clinical. Many social workers work with individuals in their families, but the extent of whole family work such as systemic family therapy undertaken by social workers is limited.

Working with service users in a group is still quite prevalent in some settings, such as probation, youth offending and mental health work, but groupwork has not been mainstream (in the UK, at least) for some time. There is a distinction between working with individuals in a group (for the convenience of bringing them all to the same place) and *groupwork*, which is the skilled use of group dynamics and group process, working with the group as a whole. Some groupwork is, therefore, better described as individual work in a group. There are some concerns in the US that generalist practice has weakened groupwork, but there are also strong arguments to support the notion that groupwork grew alongside generalist practice from the very early Settlement days that we visited in the first chapter. Generalist practice is considered in more detail in Chapter 6.

In the 1970s and 1980s in the UK, community workers would often work alongside social workers; there was a team of community workers in the area where I worked as a social worker at that time and social workers themselves would often engage in community-wide activities alongside the one-to-one work with individual clients. Community action models have a greater presence in social work in non-Western societies, such as South Africa and India but have withered in British social work.

Social work methods can usually be practised in most, if not all, of these different milieus. So, for example, task-centred family work and task-centred groupwork use the same principles as task-centred casework with individuals, but in a different milieu.

PROCESS AND OUTCOME

Social work is a profession that is oriented towards process (how things are done, the quality), and it has had to come to grips with an increasing focus on outcome (what is the product, the quantity). Of course, process and outcome are actually closely related. Family Group Conferences, mentioned earlier, are a good example of how the process of decision-making is inextricable from the decision itself.

One result of the focus on outcome is the growth of 'programmes'. These are standardised packages of work that have usually been tested and then codified into a manual of activities. The programme is delivered by social workers or other professionals, usually after they have received some training specific to the programme. An example is the 'Family Recovery Programme' aimed at supporting families trapped in a cycle of unemployment, domestic violence and poor health.

New, relatively short-lived programmes of this nature have tended to replace the established social work methods described earlier. Programmes have the advantage of being tried and tested; however, each has its own features which, though often similar to one another, are seldom sufficiently systematic or enduring for reliable comparisons to be made. This presents an obstacle to building and sustaining a systematic body of empirical knowledge.

CO-WORKING

Co-working describes a situation where two or more professionals work together directly with a service user. This can be for many reasons: a more experienced worker mentoring a new worker or student; mutual support and backup in a potentially risky situation; providing a group with a model of co-operation through co-leadership, etc. Co-working is not common and most direct social work with service users is usually a private, singular experience. This might change in the UK as part of the arrangements for supporting newly qualified social workers and continuing professional development.

A WEEK IN SOCIAL WORK

Social work is a hugely diverse activity, so it will come as no surprise that there is no 'typical week'. There are differences from one day to the next, from one setting to another and between different social workers in the same team. Nevertheless, let us try to illustrate how social workers spend their time.

Below are extracts taken from the diary notes of five *different* social workers.

MONDAY – A MENTAL HEALTH SOCIAL WORKER

Wish I could have eased myself into the week, but have a client booked in first up. Fortunately he's a good news story: a now sober alcoholic whose depression has lifted. Not surprising, given he was on a bottle of whisky a day. He's been told if he drinks again he will die. Motivation to stay off the sauce, I would imagine, though that doesn't stop some. In the afternoon I hold a best interests meeting about a client who has lost capacity to make a decision over the continued management of his finances. The meeting goes well and everyone agrees on the outcome.

TUESDAY – AN ASSESSMENT SOCIAL WORKER

Go to a child-in-need meeting at a school about a 12-year-old whose regular outbursts of anger and violence make her difficult to manage there and at home. Several agencies think it should be a child protection case because there are under-fives in the family. It does not fit the criteria and I repeat to them that procedures are not a magic pill. The last meeting decided to refer the family to an agency for direct work, but the referral was turned down. I wonder how much pain clients must suffer to receive a service.

WEDNESDAY – A SOCIAL WORKER FOR OLDER PEOPLE

Conduct a review for a man who is in a care home. He has had his leg amputated and the hospital had discharged him without a wheelchair. He tells me that he is quite happy, but that his only problem is that he can no longer cross his legs, which annoys him. Afterwards I go on a monitoring visit to a woman who had accidentally started a house fire by leaving rags on her cooker. When I try to discuss this with her she says that there has never been a fire and says that I don't know what I am talking about.

THURSDAY – A TRANSITIONS WORKER FOR YOUNG PEOPLE WITH PHYSICAL DISABILITIES

Today it's Vita. She has such severe physical disabilities that she was believed also to have profound learning disabilities. Communication technology has allowed her to show she can read and express her views. But her parents still believe that walking and talking should be priority. They won't allow the powerchair or speech simulator in the house because they make her 'lazy'. If she was under 18, I'd consider child protection proceedings. She needs her own flat.

FRIDAY – A CHILDREN AND FAMILIES SOCIAL WORKER

On duty today and work on a colleague's case where the mother has no parenting skills but wants to leave a mother and baby unit. The case has drifted, so it is hard work to catch up and ensure the child is kept at the unit while the mother leaves and we start the legal process for care proceedings. Much negotiating and persuading have to be used before the child is safe. Mental health problems seem to have dominated this week.

(With thanks to *Community Care* for permission to reproduce these five examples of social workers' weekly diaries. They appeared during 2010–11.)

Many of the themes discussed in this book emerge even in these brief notes. Thursday, to take just one example, raises issues of accountability and conflict arising from the differences between the parents' and the social worker's understanding of the client's situation. There are considerations of the law and its limitations, of labelling and reframing Vita's capacities; and the impact and potential of new technologies to empower, as well as the communication skills needed to work with or overcome the obstacles of Vita's parents' view of her world.

The diary notes above largely focus on direct work with service users, but we know that the week typically includes much time spent on other activities. Indeed, a large-scale study using social workers' diaries in the UK found that only about a quarter (26 per cent) of working time was spent in direct work with service users, a seriously shocking finding (social workers' workload survey: messages from the frontline, 2010, available at: www.dcsf.gov.uk/swtf). Case-related recording accounted for 22 per cent; case-related work in the practitioners' own agency and with other professionals a further 25 per cent of time. Finally, 26 per cent of the working week was described as 'General agency activities'. Recording, never popular, was much criticised and took longest where there were electronic systems of recording.

The working week will typically include a variety of meetings, some related to service users, others to agency matters (such as team meetings) and might include supervision with a manager and other forms of staff development.

SOCIAL WORK AND SOCIAL CARE

Social work in the UK is seen as one relatively small part of a much larger 'sector' known as social care. Social workers are often subsumed in the term 'social care professionals'. The social care workforce of about 6 million includes all those people who are employed in some capacity to meet people's social needs: in their own homes, in residential homes and in day care centres. Sometimes these staff are called carers, but this can be confusing as this same term is used for people who care informally and without payment for others, usually family members.

Social care services are locally organised and comprise a wide range of small and large organisations, some state, others private, voluntary or independent. There has been some discussion at a political level in the UK about creating a National Care Service along the lines of the National Health Service, free to all at the point of need, to provide a more co-ordinated service with less variation from location to location. The funding of such a service is the main obstacle to further development.

The recognition that health needs and social needs are closely related and require good co-ordination has led to the widespread use of the term 'heath and social care'. We will consider this in more detail towards the end of this chapter.

HOW SOCIAL WORK SERVICES ARE ORGANISED

The way in which social work services are organised is significant because the evidence from studies suggests that newly qualified social workers are quickly socialised into the culture of their employer. Social work has a tendency, therefore, to be shaped by the nature of its employment.

Social work services are organised differently from nation to nation. In developing nations non-governmental organisations (NGOs) are dominant, often international ones like Unicef. In the US the private sector is the most developed sector and social work in the health area is governed strongly by insurance eligibility. The UK has a history of public sector social work, at its pinnacle in the 1970s. In recent decades there has been more diversification, or dilution depending on your point of view. Social work has either been diluted by the loss of the large social services departments or has broadened its reach by infiltrating a wide range of sectors and settings. Either way, social work is now dispersed rather than concentrated.

The organisations that deliver social work and social care are often referred to as service providers. These providers are found in different sectors. The public sector is sometimes referred to as the first sector, the private sector the second and the voluntary sector the third.

PUBLIC SECTOR (STATUTORY)

The public sector in British social work is often described as the 'statutory' sector, a name deriving from the statutory (legal) functions that social workers and social work agencies are required to fulfil by central and local government. In France, these social workers are considered to be civil servants. Formerly in the UK, local authorities (local government or 'the council') employed the vast majority of social workers but, increasingly, the UK National Health Service directly employs social workers. The public sector accounts for the employment of an estimated 70 per cent of all social workers in the UK, a decline from around 90 per cent in the 1970s.

PRIVATE, VOLUNTARY AND INDEPENDENT (PVI) SECTORS

The private sector is composed of businesses that provide social work for profit, such as residential care homes for older people (81 per cent of all such places in England are provided by the private sector). The UK voluntary sector is non-profit and comprises well-known national charities such as NSPCC (National Society for the Prevention of Cruelty to Children) and Age UK, as well as countless small local groups.

'Voluntary' is a misleading term, as the qualified social workers that they employ are paid just as they are in the public sector. Some social workers in this 'non-statutory sector' also fulfil some statutory obligations. It should be noted that a significant proportion of the funding for voluntary organisations actually comes from the state, so that cuts to public spending affect this sector considerably. The term 'independent sector' has no clear differentiation from the private and voluntary sectors and seems to be used as a catch-all for non-public. So, the relationship between these various sectors and the terminology can be confusing.

In India the voluntary sector is known as the 'joint sector', to reflect partnerships between the state and the private sector. The state is often responsible for the initial funding, with the private sector delivering the services.

Do service users experience any difference between social workers in one sector and another? This question is difficult to answer. Certain services are not attractive to private providers because they will not make a profit; on the other hand, the public sector is highly budget-minded and rations its services accordingly. Some feel that the voluntary sector is less bound by red-tape and therefore more creative and free-thinking than the public sector; however, the voluntary sector has to spend more energy in fund-raising and sustaining projects that are dependent on short-time funding. How all of this is experienced by people who use social work services is unclear, though it should be important in formulating policy.

NEW AND DEVELOPING SHAPES

The shape and form of social work services is changing all the time, such as the rise of service user involvement in the provision of services described in the previous chapter.

'Social Care Direct' is an example of a development in the organisation of social services. This is a centralised, call centre method of responding to initial enquiries about social work and social care.

> I used to take part in a rota of social workers who, once a fortnight, spent a day 'on duty'. There would be a team of three of us ready to answer phones and see people who dropped in to the office; on a quiet day you could expect to catch up with your colleagues and case records. As well as taking some referrals that would be passed on for further work, it is true that you would also field enquiries from people wanting to know if you could help them with things like their loose chimney or the troublesome dogs next door. These 'inappropriate' contacts are seen as an inefficient use of time, and a call centre approach is designed to screen them out, so that qualified social workers only get involved when the nature of the enquiry is seen to justify it. Even so, it is perhaps a narrow view of efficiency and it is important that callers do not feel shunted around or processed, aware that the person at the other end of the phone is ticking through a set of boxes. For social workers, having time together to respond to whatever was thrown up was good for morale and team-building.

Self-help internet sites and phone contacts such as ChildLine are examples of how people can access social work, even though these services do not necessarily employ qualified social workers.

Independent social work practices, sometimes called co-operatives, social enterprises or mutuals, are a further development. At time of writing these are at the pilot stage in England, with the responsibility for over 1,000 looked-after children (children in public care) and children leaving care transferred to independent practices run by social workers in a not-for-profit capacity. The aim is to increase the workers' autonomy and therefore the likelihood of their staying and thus improve continuity for the children. Opponents fear that it is a privatisation of a public service, possibly introducing a culture of performance-related bonuses (sharing any financial surpluses amongst the staff). There are worries about future takeovers by big business as these contracts will have to be renewed and are open to undercutting competition; so they start as social enterprises but degenerate into economic enterprises. Opponents argue that ways should be found to increase the autonomy of social workers *within* the public sector.

Remote working is particularly important in areas that are geographically spread. Technologies such as video conferencing can help to support these new forms of organising social work. Hot-desking has arrived in many social work offices, with workers sharing the same desk or having to find any desk that is available. The notion of teamwork is challenged by increasing numbers of social workers expected to work from home.

HOW SOCIAL WORK SERVICES ARE BOUGHT AND SOLD

COMMISSIONING

One of the recurring themes in this book is the central place of autonomy in the notion of professional practice. A related theme is the tension between this autonomy – the power of each individual professional to decide how their time should be best used – and the desire of organisations that employ social workers to control, standardise and ration this. Add a third theme – the introduction of business practices and the market economy into public services – and we can see how social work has, in some societies, become a 'product' to buy and sell. In the jargon this is called 'commissioning' and 'providing'.

The idea lying behind the commissioning of services is that this will trigger a competitive market in social work which, in turn, will provide the people who use these services with choice and more cost-effective ways of providing them. It is especially attractive in some quarters as it is hoped to deliver cheaper services at a time when there is not the political will to pay for them.

With commissioning comes decommissioning and recommissioning. An example came to light as I was researching this book:

> A Welsh local authority withdrew funding from a local Alzheimer's group providing dementia information, advice and social support service because it was reaching 'only' 20 people. The Alzheimer's Association quickly submitted a plan with broader, reshaped services that included a network of dementia cafés and their services were recommissioned (bought again) on this basis.

This example seems to confirm the market idea of social work, one based on a pessimistic view of human nature as essentially prone to complacency and idleness and that regular market-driven jolts are needed to produce good practice.

One amongst many problems with this approach is that the process of commissioning is, itself, a cost (lawyers' and consultants' fees, procurement advice, tendering, performance monitoring and the like). Joint commissioning, when different organisations' budgets are 'pooled', is especially complex. This all needs more managers and administrators to write and rewrite bids, many of which will be unsuccessful. Change of ownership, mergers, acquisitions and insolvencies make for poor continuity for service users. It is important, then, to emphasise that the market ideology and the social ideology are at considerable odds, as we saw in Chapter 1. They are based on different beliefs about human nature but with little empirical evidence as to which approach works best in the long-term.

OUTSOURCING

The search for more cost-effective services can lead some public services to be hived off to private companies or voluntary organisations, a process known as outsourcing, as opposed to 'in-house' provision. This process has probably been greatest in social care for adults, with local authorities in the UK providing in 2011 only 19 per cent of the home care hours they funded in 2008–9.

Frequently, services can be provided more cheaply, but there are concerns that quality is sacrificed to price and that the competitive edge is gained by worsening the pay and conditions of the new employees. Outsourcing is, like commissioning, a highly politicised and ideological activity dressed up as a value-free, neutral economic strategy, with little empirical evidence to judge the longer-term consequences.

FUNDING BY RESULTS

Another possible development is funding based on the outcome of the work. This is a highly problematic area because outcomes in social work can be quite long-term, the variables are considerable (the wicked problems of page 26) and sometimes the desired goals change during, or as a consequence of, the work. The demands to set and monitor demonstrable outcomes can become the focus of the work, thus detracting from the real work. It is hard, then, to know how funding by results would work equitably in social work.

REGULATION, INSPECTION AND CONDUCT

In common with other professions, social work is subject to regulation. This is to protect the public and to retain its confidence. Systems of registration of social workers are designed to ensure that only those who are eligible to call themselves social workers can do so. Registration is sometimes known as certification, which then confers the title of social worker. In the republic of Georgia, for example, the degree in social work does not confer the professional qualification, which must be obtained from the state via an examination following the degree. Registration signals the social worker's agreement to abide by the profession's code of conduct.

Some professions have a person who speaks on behalf of the whole profession and advises the government accordingly. A chief social worker does not yet exist in the UK, though there is a call for one. Each council in Scotland has such a post, and this person has links with the chief executive and prepares annual reports on social work for the council.

ASSURING THE QUALITY OF SOCIAL WORK

It is important that people can expect a good standard of social work service no matter where they live. Arrangements for assuring the quality of social work is the business of each different country, though international codes of practice have also been developed (see Chapter 6). Complaints against individual social workers are usually investigated by the employing agency first, but professional matters can be referred to the regulator, where a conduct panel will investigate the behaviour.

Agencies are also subject to monitoring to secure standards of service. Inspectors are expected to be independent people with credibility arising from considerable knowledge and experience in their field. They need to be able to respond to individual complaints and they should have regular and personal contact with the organisations they inspect, including contact with a sample of the people who use the social work services. There are some fundamental questions about inspection that are still in need of a coherent response: should inspection take place routinely or only when there are concerns and perceived risks? At what levels should inspection take place?

As noted earlier in this chapter, social work is seen as part of the broader realm of social care in the UK, and these overall standards are monitored by the Care Quality Commission (CQC), with Ofsted responsible for the inspection and regulation of services for children and young people. However, it is one thing to set standards and another to assess whether and how they are being met. Performance assessment is a controversial area, with polarised views about whether it should refer 'downwards', with local account-ability to the people who use the services, or 'upwards', meeting central targets set by government. Social work values would suggest downwards accountability, though the mechanics for this are not straightforward and some feel strongly that there is a need for nation-ally published data that allow comparisons of the performance of different councils and organisations.

The trends that have created a market for social services have also led to a market in quality-assurance regimes, with private consultancy firms blossoming, whilst the documentation to assess performance becomes onerous and complex. New kinds of social work provi-sion, such as the independent social work practices discussed earlier, will test existing forms of regulation and accountability.

In addition to inspection and assessment it is important that knowl-edge about good and excellent social work practice is systematically collected, evaluated and disseminated. We will consider this in more detail in the next chapter. For now, let us note that the Social

Care Institute for Excellence (Scie) is charged with identifying and spreading best practice across social services in parts of the UK. An influential 'Learning Network' for social work and social policy (SWAP) was abolished by the UK Coalition government in 2011.

WORKFORCE ORGANISATIONS

We will explore training, education and professional development for social work in the next chapter, but note here that the development of the broader social care workforce in the UK is overseen by two organisations, Skills for Care for adult services, and the Children's Workforce Development Council for children's services (the latter transfers to the Department for Education). These organisations are tasked with improving training and workforce standards.

SANCTIONS

What sanctions are available to be used against social workers and agencies that do not fulfil the required standards?

As noted, most countries have mechanisms to regulate social workers whose conduct causes concern. For instance:

- A social worker caught with traces of magic mushrooms and half an ecstasy tablet received a 'three year admonishment', largely because he failed to notify his employer and the regulator.
- A social worker was found to have failed to carry out statutory (legally required) visits to five children, though the panel took into account her large caseload and problems with management.
- Failure to report a colleague's behaviour can also lead to action.

Serious breaches can result in suspension from practising, removal from the register, and even prosecution.

The misconduct of individual social workers is often entangled with the chaotic circumstances of their agency. The latter can be a mitigating factor and 'systemic failings' are often cited in the inquiries that follow calamitous events. There is a voluntary code for social service agencies in the UK, with calls to make this legally enforceable.

What should a social worker do if they feel that their agency is not supporting good practice? Professional bodies representing social work usually have guidance if professionals face substandard agency practices, but no-one should pretend this is easy. (See the section on Whistleblowing on page 55.)

RELATIONS WITH THE NEIGHBOURS

MULTIPROFESSIONAL WORK

Social work borders and overlaps many other professions and there has always been a need to work closely with these neighbours: teachers, doctors, police, lawyers, probation officers, health visitors, occupational therapists, community workers, community mental health workers, psychiatrists, residential workers, housing workers and many others. Increasingly, social workers have found themselves employed in teams composed of different professionals, in multiprofessional teams.

What does social work bring to these teams? In a team working with people with learning difficulties (sometimes referred to as intellectual disabilities), the non-social work professionals were asked what they thought was the unique social work contribution to the work. They listed the following:

- focusing on social rather than medical models of disability (see pages 18–19);
- a holistic perspective;
- a strategic approach to organisations;
- the co-ordinating abilities of social workers;
- a certain quality of relationship with service users which was somehow 'closer'.

One of the non-social work members said, 'What is valuable is [social work] just having a broader, all-encompassing view of the community and the people and what's out there. A much wider picture than some of the other disciplines.'

Using a contrast approach in this way can be enlightening, i.e. investigating a phenomenon, in this case the nature of social work, by asking those who are outside social work.

HEALTH – LIVING WITH A POWERFUL NEIGHBOUR

The most powerful of all social work's neighbours is health. In the UK the National Health Service is a huge employer and a highly significant part of the nation's identity; medicine is a major player and health is a highly politicised area. Social work is tiny by contrast. Social care as a whole is bigger than health in terms of numbers, but there is no single National Care Service and its employees are poorly paid. Social care is significantly less powerful than medicine; for example, for every £1 spent on research in social work and social care, it is estimated that £17 is spent in health research, and this does not include pharmaceutical research. In 2011 it was announced that the UK National Institute for Health and Clinical Excellence (NICE) would relieve its social care equivalent (Scie) of some of its role in developing and disseminating good practice in social care. At the same time, the regulatory functions of the General Social Care Council (GSCC) will be subsumed within the Health Professions Council (HPC).

Social work increasingly has been joined to health. This is curious, because social workers are as likely to have contact with many other professions as they are with healthcare practitioners. In my own practice I rarely needed to work closely with a nurse, other than community mental health nurses as they were known (a tiny proportion of all nurses), whilst I had regular contact with probation officers, lawyers, housing workers, community workers, teachers and the police.

Social work has had a tendency to be caught in the coat-tails of the powerful fashion of the time, in this case health. This trend has also been evident in the movement of the discipline of social work away from sociology and social policy departments and into faculties of health and social care, even though the social sciences as a discipline are closer to social work than are the health sciences.

RELATIONS WITH OTHER PROFESSIONS

Most of the social work services that involve children and families are now organisationally linked to education services in England. Children's services departments have been formed by removing children's work from former social services departments and locating it within former education departments. This has been driven by an attempt to integrate services for children and families, but one result has been that many social work services for children are managed by people with no social work background.

The effect of the organisational retreat of social work from its own home base and into teams hosted by other professions (health, education, youth justice, etc.) has yet to be thoroughly researched. Success could mean that the social work ethos described in Chapter 1 has a wider acceptance and has influenced other professions; failure will have led the profession to become marginalised and less confident of its future role.

INTEGRATING SERVICES

The desire to promote 'joined up' services, where the boundary between the various professions is invisible to the people using them, has led to a belief in the value of integrating services. We saw in the last section how children's social work has been integrated with local educational services. Inquiries into tragedies such as child deaths regularly point to the poor co-ordination of services as a contributing factor.

Decisions about whether a person has an overnight stay in hospital (health) or receives support at home in the community (social care) are too often made on the basis of which budget pays. 'Pooled budgets', into which more than one organisation contributes, are seen as one way to support practitioners who want the basis for these decisions to be the service user's needs rather than the most available budget. However, this kind of joint funding accounted for only 3.4 per cent of health and social care funding in the UK in 2009.

One response to co-ordinating services is to have a lead professional (a key worker) for the service user and their family. This person may or may not be the social worker, but takes responsibility for liaising between the various organisations and professionals so that the service user is not passed from pillar to post.

As with many of the notions that we have been exploring in this book, integrating services is an act of faith rather than evidence-based. Poorly supervised professionals in an integrated department are, one could suppose, less likely to provide a seamless service than professionals who are confident in their own role and develop their own mechanisms to co-ordinate their work with other similarly confident, well-supported professionals. We will develop this further in the next chapter when we explore interprofessional learning.

IN CONCLUSION

In this chapter we have explored social work as a profession, the profile of the workforce, its working conditions and what social workers do when they meet with service users. We have established the central place of autonomy, accountability and authority in the notion of professional practice and the difficulties of balancing these elements with the expectations of common standards of practice and the need to regulate and inspect the outcomes of social work. The chapter has reviewed the economics and organisation of social work services, set in the broader context of social care and other professional groups.

FURTHER READING

V. Cree (ed.), *Becoming a Social Worker*, London: Routledge, 2003.
Thirteen stories of journeys into social work practice, management and education, aiming to make social work more visible.

P. Marsh and M. Doel, *The Task-centred Book*, London: Routledge/Community Care, 2006.
A comprehensive overview of task-centred social work, one of the few 'home-grown' methods. Plenty of examples from the direct work of task-centred practitioners illustrate the book.

W. J. Reid, *The Task Planner*, New York: Columbia University Press, 2000.
A rare, comprehensive collection of the research data deriving from one particular social work method.

S. Rogowski, *Social Work: The Rise and Fall of a Profession*, Bristol: The Policy Press, 2010.
A committed, radical critique of British social work with an interesting historical sweep. It is written by a practitioner with many decades' experience.

SOME RELATED WEBLINKS

www.basw.co.uk British Association of Social Workers.
www.childline.org.uk enables confidential talk about issues troubling or concerning children, with message boards and telephone lines and access to a counsellor.

www.communitycare.co.uk/blogs/diary-of-a-social-worker.
www.dh.gov.uk Department of Health.
www.education.gov.uk Department for Education.
www.gscc.org.uk General Social Care Council.
www.hpc-uk.org Health Professions Council.
https://knowledgehub.local.gov.uk Local Government Association.
www.skillsforcare.org.uk Skills for Care (workforce development council).
http://socialcaredirect.org Social Care Direct.
www.socialworkers.org National (US) Association of Social Workers.

REFERENCES

Smith, R. 'High caseloads hitting practice', *Community Care*, 9/9/10: 5.

Community Care (2010), 'Dress for success', 9/12/10: 28.

Community Care (2010), 'Social care staff face pay freeze and poorer working conditions', 9/12/10: 4–5.

Community Care (2011), 'Poll results: How would you react to a 5% pay cut?', 3/3/11: 13.

5

A DISCIPLINE OR A SKILL; AN EDUCATION OR A TRAINING
HOW SOCIAL WORKERS LEARN THEIR PRACTICE

In this chapter we consider social work as a field of study, learn about social work skills and discover how social workers are educated.

A DISCIPLINE

Social work has had a place in university faculties for many decades, with training and education starting in the UK and US at the beginning of the twentieth century. Sometimes it constitutes its own school or institute (especially in the US), but more often it is subsumed with other disciplines, such as sociological studies or, increasingly in the UK, with health professionals. As a 'soft' science with a strong practical orientation and a history of borrowing from other disciplines such as sociology and psychology, social work has had a struggle to establish itself as a discipline in its own right.

Social work is eclectic, borrowing from various sources. This is fine but it needs to be systematic and considered, not an attraction to the latest box of intellectual fireworks. The most pressing concern for the profession is to build, and build on, a careful construction of cumulative, usable knowledge with social work practice as the foundation. In fact, social work's holistic perspective puts it in a strong position when it comes to the fashion for intellectual 'sandpits' in which theorists and practitioners from a wide variety of different disciplines come together to cross boundaries in the hope of coming up with innovative, rounded theories and practices.

SOCIAL WORK RESEARCH

The nature of social work research is contested in the way that the profession itself is and the disputes in social work reflect those in the larger research community, particularly around the nature of evidence.

Should social work researchers emphasise objectivity and establish strict scientific tests that aim to control the different factors, 'the variables'?

> In this empirical paradigm we might study two social work teams with a similar composition and a similar demographic. We might introduce some kind of change with one of the teams (e.g. train them in a new method of practice or develop a new recording system) and then measure what, if any, impact this change has.

Randomised controlled trials of this kind are dominant in the medical sciences and are often considered highest value, but critics in the social sciences argue that the variables are too great for these methods to be useful and that there can be insurmountable ethical issues – and that they are expensive, too.

Should we, then, recognise the messiness of social work and rely on methods that are described as qualitative? These methods seek to tell a more detailed story, usually of a smaller landscape, with a belief that there is no single 'truth', no proven objective facts, and that realities are socially constructed.

Taking our example of the two social work teams above, a qualitative researcher might construct a case study of each to reflect their respective experiences and to understand the meanings each team attributes to its work, perhaps contrasting the two.

Critics of this approach question what benefit is derived from knowledge that is so case specific and cannot be generalised to other situations. However, this polarisation between what are loosely described as quantitative and qualitative approaches is false. It is perfectly possible to mix these methods, so that the subjective nature of truth is recognised whilst the search for proven facts, or at least likelihoods, is not abandoned.

If we look at what is most distinctive about social work research, it is probably the central place of service users, less as research subjects and increasingly as research partners. The value of research is often measured by its impact, but the question is *impact on whom?* The social work discipline emphasises the impact of a research study on those who experience social work, rather than, say, the number of times the study is referenced by other researchers in academic articles. Indeed, social work journals have relatively modest international rankings.

The resources for social work research are relatively limited and often prescribed so that research is often tailored to the immediate short-term needs of those commissioning the research rather than large-scale social work research. This relatively piecemeal approach has made it difficult to establish a baseline (i.e. what is actually happening now) on which to build future policy and practice.

DOCTORAL SOCIAL WORK

The need for social work academics to have a credible professional background means that many progress to academic life later in their careers. A trade-off between professional and scholarly experience means a majority of senior academics in the UK have not studied at doctoral level. Even so, social work at doctoral level is strengthening. In the US and in many continental European countries it is not possible to teach at certain levels at a university without a PhD, though research at this level is constrained in Germany by the fact that social work is only taught at institutions which cannot award PhDs.

In addition to the traditional research-led PhD, two other routes are sometimes possible. First, a PhD by publication is open to candidates who have substantial publications. They can gather a themed sample of their publications and submit them for examination, along with a critical commentary of the research that underpins the publications. The publications must be judged to be of doctoral standard and the candidate has a viva with examiners in the same manner as a 'taught' or traditional PhD. A second route is the Professional Doctorate which has some taught elements, such as research methods, and is usually part-time and tailored to practitioners and managers. In the US the DSW (Doctor in Social Work) is considered the professional doctoral degree, and the PhD in social work is seen as the research or academic one. There are few DSW programmes.

Doctoral level research in social work is of great significance to the future development of social work as an academic discipline as well as building knowledge for, from and about practice.

EVIDENCE-BASED PRACTICE

Practitioners are expected to keep up with the latest developments in research in order to base their practice on the best evidence available. This notion is summed up as 'evidence-based practice'. However, the notion is not as straightforward as it seems and the complexities are linked to our earlier discussion of the different approaches to research. The perspectives of researchers, practitioners and service users can and do differ as to what constitutes a successful outcome for social work, and this raises the question, *whose* evidence?

'Evidence' can be experienced as somehow distant from the messiness of practice and not especially useful for day-to-day social work practice. *Practice-based evidence* turns the notion on its head to suggest that evidence should be derived first and foremost from practice. In a discipline that has a practice, like social work, there is a preference for research that has obvious practical applications; yet social work practice is so shaped by its context and so specific to each circumstance that it is difficult to draw practice prescriptions from research evidence that can be meaningful to each particular situation.

Although practitioners are exhorted to use evidence-based practice, the example set by policymakers and government too frequently highlights ways in which inconvenient truths are quietly shelved in favour of pragmatism or ideology. This can create cynicism but should not in itself discredit an evidence-based approach. It is critical that social work continues to build its own body of practice-based evidence, one that is meaningful to the people who practise social work and who experience it.

EVALUATION

Research is often described as differing from evaluation in that the former builds new knowledge through critical and scientific enquiry whilst the latter assesses the effectiveness of existing knowledge and experience. In practice the two shade into one another and, apart from meeting different criteria for research funding and research ethics, the distinctions are not significant.

Like all professions, social work has a responsibility to find out how effective it is. Some practice methods have evaluative mechanisms built into the method itself:

> The careful recording of problems, goals, tasks and reviews that occurs as part of task-centred social work, introduced in the previous chapter, provides a document of the effectiveness, or otherwise, of the method. In addition to reviews at the beginning of each session, a final evaluation asks a number of standardised questions that indicate progress and service users' understanding of the process and their feelings about it. The method is not confined to individualised casework but can be used with groups and organisations and can measure changes in people's understanding of structural issues as well as personal ones.

Evaluative methods that are integral to practice methods, such as the one just described, are more likely to be used by social workers because they avoid imposing an additional layer of work and are more meaningful to the service users themselves. External evaluations are likely to be seen as tangential to the main work, but they are perceived as independent and therefore more credible. Finding ways to corroborate evidence that is gathered by 'insider researchers' (i.e. people researching their own practice) is important, a process known as triangulation.

THEORY AND PRACTICE

Take a cup of oil, add it to a cup of vinegar and shake vigorously. For a while the two will emulsify but, left to itself, quite soon the mix will separate out. This is how many social workers think about theory and practice: with tremendous will you can integrate them for a while, but their natural state is separation, one floating above the other.

In fact, social workers theorise all the time in their work and from it. If these pet theories become generally accepted they develop into *practice wisdom*. This is based on repeated experiences which generalise into working theories and hypotheses:

> That middle children are more likely to become young offenders; that a move into residential care adds to the confusion of someone with dementia; that it is harmful to a black child's development to be placed with a white adoptive family.

Some practice wisdom is contested within the profession, some has formal research that supports or contradicts it (or does both at the same time). The point is that social work practice 'mixes' with theory all the time, though it is frequently implicit and not recognised.

Formal theory, that is theory with a capital letter and perhaps an 'ism', like Marxism, often provides a comprehensive explanation for a set of circumstances but not necessarily a prescription for how to use the theory in practice. This missing link is what makes theory seem alien to many practitioners. When I was training as a social worker I was much taken with the anti-psychiatry movement and the theories of R.D. Laing. When I first started to practise social work I found Laing's theories powerful and convincing as explanations but they gave me no idea at all what to *do* when sitting in somebody's living room.

Social work theory needs to be able to explain the world from a broad ecological perspective (systems theories have often proved useful as well as feminist perspectives, as we saw in Chapter 1) *and* also to provide guidance about what to do with these explanations. We saw in the last chapter how task-centred social work is based on theories about learning and also on systems theory. It has an explicit methodology that helps practitioners to put these theories into practice *and* the experience of this practice contributes to the theory-building. At their best, theory and practice are cyclical, the one supporting the other.

SOCIAL WORK SKILLS

Do social workers have skills that others do not have and, if so, what are they? The short answer is that social work does not have a single, unique skill, but that the set of skills comprising social work is distinctive and specific to social work.

These skills are marked by the fact that they are so wide-ranging. A list can never be exhaustive, but here is an attempt at some of the main skills:

To use and generate theory and research, develop a critical understanding of policy and challenge injustice; to observe, listen, communicate and make balanced judgements through the medium of interviews; to plan, organise, strategise and manage resources; to engage with task and purpose over time; to convey empathy and understanding; to develop and explore hypotheses; to question, make and communicate decisions and the reasoning behind them and to record this; to provide direct help, guidance and material assistance; give support and care; offer interpretations and explanations; model partnership, negotiate with other agencies and professionals, advocate, challenge and confront; deal with aggression and manage professional boundaries; evaluate effectiveness, reflect on practice and look after own well-being; transfer learning from one situation to another and pursue professional development.

Social workers deploy all of these skills in a great variety of settings, contexts and milieux – with individuals, families, groups, communities and organisations. The breadth of both the skill and the setting is one of the unusual aspects of social work and sums up what it means to work with 'the person in their environment'. In the UK these skills are codified to some extent in occupational standards and a framework of professional capabilities (see conclusion of chapter for weblink).

Let us take just a few social work skills and explore them in a little more detail.

ASSERTIVENESS

Social workers need to be able to protect themselves if they are to be in a position to help others, like the pre-flight safety demonstration to fix your own oxygen mask before helping others. Their ability to do this depends on the extent to which they feel that power lies within them or outside them, sometimes described as an internal or external locus of control. The powerlessness that many service users feel in their lives can find itself mirrored in the feelings of social workers themselves.

Making changes, whether this is service users or social workers, requires time to explore alternatives and take action, with the risks of rejection and failure, and a belief that change is possible. Notions of empowerment and emancipation are meaningless without assertiveness, which gives people the power to challenge submissiveness and self-defeating beliefs.

Assertive social workers can say no to unacceptable workloads and can defend good practice in their agencies, avoiding complicity with malpractice and lowering tolerance of negligent behaviour such as partner professionals failing to carry through agreed actions. For instance, disrespectful treatment of older people in a hospital by health care workers should be seen by social workers as something to challenge, not something to manage.

Unassertive behaviour has a direct, negative impact on the lives of people whom social work is charged to protect.

SELF-DISCLOSURE

All professionals regularly grapple with decisions about how much or how little to disclose to the people with whom they work. They are asked if they are married, have children, work with other people in this kind of situation, etc., and they have to decide how to respond. The easy answer is not to take any risks by disclosing nothing. However, this carries risks, too, that opportunities to advance the relationship with the service user are lost. Judging the fine balance between distance and warmth makes social work interesting and challenging. In almost all circumstances the complexities should lead to a response of 'it depends' and the capable social worker is the one who can articulate what the 'it' is.

In addition to their personal biographies, social workers might be asked about their beliefs. In some situations social workers must decide how much to disclose about the way a decision has been taken and the extent to which they agree or disagree with it. It is not only politicians who have to grapple with the consequences of collective responsibility.

What social workers really want to avoid is generating the kind of feedback that led a foster parent to describe her contacts with the child's social worker thus:

'Her phone calls always end up being about her problems – illness, family issues, broken windscreen wipers'.

(*Guardian Weekend*, 27/11/10: 23)

It is one thing to show your human side and another to be a burden or an ineffectual victim.

RECORDING

Recording social work interventions is necessary to satisfy legal and administrative requirements and to provide continuity of service. Compiled together with the service user, records can be a powerful, participative tool that is integral to the social work intervention.

The development of electronic data has led to increasing standardisation of forms to collect information (such as the Common Assessment Framework in children's social work), but we should remind ourselves that the whole activity of recording is a significant part of the *professional* task. Within broad parameters set by the agency, social workers should use professional judgement to decide what is to be recorded and how. The challenge is to recapture the professional skill of recording whilst harnessing the power that modern electronic data collection provides. At the heart of this is the tension between professional discretion and standardised information (to determine people's eligibility for services and to cover the agency in any future legal action).

Recording has never been a welcome task, but it is evident that it occupies more time that it used to, certainly in British social work, detracting from face-to-face work with service users. I used to speak directly into a dictaphone immediately following a meeting with a client (often in the car afterwards), with the transcript then typed up by a secretary, so the recording was immediate and brief. Very old-tech, but surprisingly efficient. Laptops could be used to the same effect. A local authority in north-east England issues its social workers with tablet PCs (similar to iPads), with handwriting recognition software, to make their recordings on the spot when appropriate.

As we learned in the first chapter, documenting social work is important for the development of the profession. It is important to find ways to use the information available in social workers' *portfolios* of practice to develop practice. We will return to portfolios later.

NEW SKILLS AND NEW TECHNOLOGIES

Many service user groups use social media to build support networks. An example is netbuddy.org.uk that connects carers of children with learning disabilities. Interactive virtual environments are available to prepare young people in care for independent living and there are many dedicated websites for different service user groups.

There is some resistance to the use of social media by social workers themselves because of perceived difficulties with confidentiality, reinforced by cases such as internet bullying that have been prominent in the media. However, groups can restrict membership to those who have been approved. Some agencies have restrictive policies about the flow of information, yet those agencies that embrace the new possibilities will be developing services that are more in touch with the lives of their service users. Some chief executives and local councillors are writing blogs and using Twitter to communicate with their local communities, and social media could help social workers to share good practice, not just locally but internationally.

Sometimes the challenge is to support old skills with new technologies. For example, two of the most basic skills are to be at a place at the time you said you would be and to do what you promise to do. The social worker who can use a personal organiser to assist punctuality and reliability has a great advantage.

IMAGINATION

Imagination might be more an attribute than a skill, but the ability to conjure a different set of circumstances or to place yourself somewhere else is an asset in many ways: the imagination to empathise with someone else's situation at an individual level, and the imagination to think outside the usual constraints when working for solutions. Imagination is a key factor in the nebulous notion of reflection, allowing alternative ways of looking at ourselves and others to create different meanings and mindsets.

REFLECTIVE PRACTICE

It is generally thought that professional practice benefits when there is the opportunity and the ability to reflect on that practice. Social workers need to reflect both *in* actual practice and then, subsequently, back *on* their practice. Reflection is a skill and, therefore, can be learned. However, there has been an uncritical acceptance of the value of reflection and further research is needed to establish what it is and whether it does indeed improve practice.

COMPETENCE APPROACH

People who use social work services want their social workers to be competent at their jobs. Managers in social work agencies want practitioners fit for the job. Concerns about the abilities of some social workers, especially highlighted by public enquiries into child deaths, powered the development of the competence approach to training social workers. In this approach social work is divided into key roles which spell out what social workers should be able to do, and further subdivided into 'performance indicators' which aim to show whether they are achieving competence.

An example of a competence is to be able 'to support individuals to represent their needs, views and enhance well-being'. In the UK this is one of six key roles that social workers are expected to perform. Their equivalents in the US are the ten core competencies outlined in the Council on Social Work Education's Educational Policy and Accreditation Standards (EPAS). An example of a competence from these standards is to be able to 'respond to contexts that shape practice'. This can be spelled out further, for instance that social workers are active in responding to evolving organisational, community and societal contexts.

Critics of the competence approach note that it is not possible to cover all eventualities (the list of competences is potentially limitless) and that this partial approach loses sight of the bigger picture, like a microbiologist who thinks that the quality of a cake can be estimated by putting crumbs of it under the microscope rather than eating it.

HOLISTIC APPROACH

Brain surgeons need to be highly skilled and the required competences take years to develop, but these competences are relatively specific, easily observed and the results are obvious. Competence in social work is more difficult to pinpoint because it is a holistic practice; that is, social work concerns itself with the whole individual in their social context. It is perhaps the most situation-specific profession, so that what is seen as competent in one place and time might not be seen as such in another.

The polarisation of the competence and holistic approaches is another example of unhelpful dualism; i.e. a belief that it has to be either A or B, not A and B. Of course social workers need to be competent at their work; and part of this competence is the ability to understand the reality of a service user's life *as a whole*, and to work with the many different levels that have an impact.

As an example, let us consider social work and HIV-AIDS. Social workers support individual HIV-positive people to manage the disorder, but they also work with their families to promote acceptance and with the wider community to counter the social stigma of AIDS. It is part of the social work role to fight ignorance at the highest political levels – for example, beliefs that AIDS is not caused by the HIV virus. This is a holistic perspective and it requires competences at many different levels.

EDUCATION AND TRAINING

Another dualism is that between social work as an education (a grounding in a discipline within the social sciences) and social work as a training (learning how to do it). Of course, both are essential. A social work education provides the necessary foundation upon which the newly graduated social worker can develop abilities to practise ethically, effectively and responsively. Training students to 'do a section 47 enquiry' before they are educated to understand the complexities of people, social relationships and legal frameworks, makes no sense. (Section 47 of the Children Act 1989 requires a local authority in England and Wales to carry out an Enquiry where there is information that a child has suffered or is likely to suffer significant harm.)

SOCIAL WORK EDUCATION

Social work education is grounded in the liberal arts and these provide the intellectual basis for the professional curriculum. Increasingly, social work is a graduate profession, meaning social workers must have a degree before they are able to practise. Social work is offered as an undergraduate subject for study for three or four years at a university or college offering higher education degrees. Social work is also offered as a Master's level award by progressing from the BSW to the MSW or, in some cases, for students whose first degree is in another subject but who wish to train for social work.

Social work degree courses are offered by 103 institutions in the UK, where there was a record 60,000 applicants for about 6,000 places for the 2010 intake of full-time undergraduate courses. Students are selected using a combination of academic attainment, a personal written statement, and interview (individual, group or both). Service users are involved in all aspects of social work education in the UK, including the selection process. In the US there are more than 660 accredited social work degree programmes.

As we will see later, there is an emphasis on learning in placements settings, and this has been in evidence since the early days (see page 19).

STUDENT SOCIAL WORKERS

There were 16,641 social work students registered in England in 2011, 1,897 in Scotland, 840 in Wales and 566 in Northern Ireland. Over 31,000 full-time social work students (and over 5,200 part-time ones) were enrolled on BSW programmes in the US in 2009; and 30,000 full-time and over 17,700 part-time for MSW programmes (statistics from the Council on Social Work Education website).

Social work attracts mature students as well as those coming straight from school and the average age of social work students at entry in the UK is 30 years old. Undergraduate social work students coming to university straight from school can be surprised that expectations are different for students on professional courses. Standards for the behaviour of social work students are set high, especially when they are in placement settings. The gender imbalance in social work that was noted in Chapter 3 is reflected in the student population; women make up 84 per cent of British social work students.

DROP OUT

Social work in the UK has a 1 in 7 drop out rate, similar to other professional degree courses (the 2008–9 figures were 2,170 out of 14,550 students). This is different from the failure rate (3.4 per cent), as some students leave the course voluntarily, perhaps because they do not feel that social work is right for them, or for personal, economic and health reasons. Also included in these figures are students who will be returning to study, sometimes called an intermission. Social work training courses act as gate-keepers to the profession and, ultimately, a protection for service users. There is always regret when a student's future career is terminated, with all the attendant feelings of failure, but it is paramount to protect the people with whom students would be working as future social workers.

FUNDING AND COSTS

The funding of students' study is a political issue and one that arouses controversy. The funding of professional courses such as social work is especially contentious as it costs more, in terms of staff–student ratios, to provide training for the professions and these students know that they will earn only modest salaries with which to pay off student debts. If a society desires public servants such as social workers, so the argument runs, then it needs to make sure there is adequate financial support to train and educate them.

In recent years bursaries have been available to cushion the costs of a social work education. Different parts of the UK are finding their own solutions to these issues – and the funding of social work students varies widely around the world. Suffice it to say that the dedication and commitment of people wishing to become social workers will stretch only so far and that the case for continued financial help is strong, at least for modestly paid professional groups like social workers.

BECOMING A SOCIAL WORKER

Social work is a demanding subject of study because it requires people who are 'all-rounders': intellectual, emotional and interpersonal abilities are needed in roughly equal measure. This combination of talents is relatively unusual and often underestimated.

THE SOCIAL WORK CURRICULUM

A curriculum is a statement of how knowledge, values and skills will be learned and assessed in order to become a successful social worker. In the UK the ownership of the curriculum is shared between social work professional bodies, universities, government departments, regulatory bodies and service user educators. The standards developed by various regulatory bodies must be adhered to.

In Chapter 1 we reproduced the syllabus from 1908 for a 'training for social and philanthropic work' at the University of Birmingham. Below, a century later, is the curriculum on a typical three-year UK undergraduate degree (from Sheffield Hallam University, England).

First year
Psychosocial Studies 1 and 2
Foundations of Social Work
Using Knowledge and Evidence to Support Study and Practice
Introduction to Interprofessional Practice
Values and Anti-Oppressive Practice
Social Work Law and Processes
The People We Work With
Readiness to Practice and Safeguarding

Second year
Practice Learning 1 (Placement)
Assessment, Planning, Intervention and Review
Global Issues in Social Work Practice
Developing Collaborative Practice
Using and Evaluating Evidence to Inform Practice

Third year
Law for Social Work
Values, Ethics and Dilemmas
Practice Learning 2 (Placement)
Generating and Evaluating Evidence for Practice
Capable Collaborative Working

Social work degree courses are divided into modules (in some countries these are called courses though, confusingly, in the UK the whole programme is often referred to as 'the course'). The proportion of time 'on placement' in social work agencies varies from country to country but in the UK it is approximately half.

The distinction is sometimes made between the explicit and the implicit curriculum. The former is the programme's formal educational structure, designed with specific aims in mind. The latter refers to the environment that supports the explicit curriculum, such as admissions policies that widen access to disadvantaged groups, participation by students and service users in the governance of the programme, proper allocation of resources for student support, fair termination procedures, and a commitment to diversity.

UNDERGRADUATE AND POSTGRADUATE

In the US there is a clear distinction between the undergraduate BSW (Bachelor level) and the postgraduate MSW (Master's level). The BSW curriculum prepares its graduates for generalist practice whilst the MSW prepares for advanced practice with an element of specialisation (called 'a concentration'). In the UK, the *qualifying* (professional) elements of the Bachelor's and Master's degrees in social work are the same, measured by the same criteria and to the same standard. The distinction between undergraduate and postgraduate is generally only made in the standard of students' academic work.

This line between academic and practical work is not clear-cut and a pass in both elements is required. There is usually an 'exit' award for those students who might succeed with their academic assignments but fail with their placements; otherwise, an academically sound but professionally inept student could leave university with nothing to show for their time and effort. However, it is not possible to achieve the professional qualification without the academic success.

FULL-TIME, PART-TIME AND WORK-BASED

There are different routes to the social work qualification. The traditional one is as a full-time student based in a university or college. However, social work has developed other routes to include students whose circumstances make full-time study impossible.

Part-time routes enable students to continue with family responsibilities and remain economically active. Some routes allow the student to continue in work, with the study shaped around the worker-student's workplace, known as 'grow your own' schemes. Although they have tremendous advantages in terms of convenience and finance, there are concerns about a clash between the student role and the employee role, with the 'student' possibly not achieving sufficient independence from their agency. Some schemes aim to overcome this drawback by making reciprocal arrangements with neighbouring local authorities so that students can have a wider variety of placement and a more detached perspective on their workplace.

DISTANCE, FLEXIBLE, OPEN, VIRTUAL AND MOBILE LEARNING

In addition to the routes described above there are also different *modes* by which to study social work. The terms *distance*, *open*, *flexible* and *virtual* are sometimes used interchangeably, but there are distinctions. Distance learning is, as the term implies, conducted away from the central site of education to accommodate people who cannot attend in person, perhaps because of geography or restricted mobility.

Flexible learning is used to emphasise learning that is personally tailored around the individual student. So, it might indicate a combination of distance and on-site learning, but it can also refer to a mix of teaching and learning methods that we explore next. This combination of approaches and methods can be called *blended learning*.

Open learning describes less the place of learning and more the style and method – the *pedagogy*. An example of a formal pedagogy is 'talk and chalk', when students sit in rows listening to their teacher talking and writing on a board. An informal pedagogical style is the seminar or workshop, in which students take a more active part in their learning, guided by the tutor or workshop leader, but often making their own preparations and taking their own initiative in small groups. This is sometimes referred to as *adult learning*, though children equally benefit from and enjoy this approach. This active, participative learning is apparent in a method called problem-based learning, when students are asked to work together to explore a theme or situation and to advance strategies to help solve or work with the problem.

The power of simulation has long been known in some training environments, such as airline pilots who can learn how to manage a damaged aircraft without having to put lives or expensive machinery at risk. For practical and economic reasons the virtual learning environment (VLE) has been less developed in social work, though this is changing. Simulation permits standardised situations to be used repeatedly, without putting real people at risk or discomfort. Once created it is very economic. However, the sophistication of human interaction and the chemistry of social situations is very difficult to achieve in a VLE and can feel inauthentic. Even so, if we look at virtual worlds their success comes not from the recreation of this reality but from the availability of another reality where people can practise being another self or an alternative side of their self (one such is called *Second Life*). This is the best way forward for virtual learning in social work, to provide opportunities to rehearse other possibilities, not to attempt a faithful recreation of reality: 'reality' is what placements are for.

The technology of pedagogies, that is, the ways students are taught and can learn, continues apace with *mobile learning*, using mobile phones, iPods and the like.

INTERPROFESSIONAL LEARNING

If different professions are to work well together there is a belief that they should be educated together. Many social work programmes in the UK include a module of learning in which students from different professional courses learn together. Occasionally a whole programme is interprofessional and leads to jointly qualified practitioners: for example, practitioners who are qualified both as social workers and as nurses in the field of learning disability.

The combination of students who are brought together reflects the way in which the particular university organises its faculties – commonly healthcare and social work together. Given the range of other professionals who work in close proximity with social workers – lawyers, teachers, psychologists, etc. – the dominance of health groupings is disproportionate. Moreover, there is one group of health workers that is frequently absent: doctors.

Putting people of different professions in the same room could reinforce prejudices and stereotyping, so it is important that the teaching and learning methods are carefully designed to enable differences and similarities to be understood and respected.

There is a degree of political expediency in the move to aggregate or disaggregate professional education. For example, social work used to be highly integrated with probation in the UK and the two professions trained together, so that probation officers were also qualified social workers. This interprofessional partnership was forcibly split in England in the 1990s, when probation education was separated completely from social work education.

PLACEMENTS AND PRACTICE LEARNING

Placement in a practical setting is a central component of social work education. Students in the UK spend about half of the programme in practice settings, sometimes called fieldwork, but in Russia, for instance, it is frequently less than 10 per cent. Placements usually have a big impact on students, remembered in ways that class-based learning is not. It is nearly forty years since my own placements, but I remember them well: one in a Probation Office, then a residential placement in the adolescent unit of a psychiatric hospital, and finally a placement in the social services department of a port city. It is not unusual to hear social workers clearly recollect, as I can, the clients and colleagues with whom they worked during their placements.

Placements are frequently demanding and inexperienced students can find them a daunting prospect. Unlike the class setting where it is possible to snuggle into the crowd, the one-to-one focus on a placement allows no such cover. Any communication problems become starkly evident on placement, and a range of other difficulties, such as dyslexia, might not be revealed until then. Fortunately, the placement provides, or should provide, individual tuition and supervision, and a recognition that this is a place for *learning* – that students are students and not novice practitioners.

A general shortage of placements in the UK led to the use of new sites, such as schools, prisons, community groups and private foster agencies. At its best, this enables students to be more experimental and innovative and to understand social work as a broader activity than procedure-driven practice. At its worst, students are left floundering, trying to understand where 'the social work' is in these placements and worried that they will not be able to find evidence that they have achieved the necessary standards for social work. The key to transforming the worst to the best is, as we will explore later, the role of supervision.

SIGNATURE PEDAGOGY

The way in which social work placements are conceptualised has undergone a significant transformation. Fieldwork used to be perceived as the place where students put the theory they learned in college into practice. In fact, more often than not, field practice seemed rather remote and distinct from the academic work in class, a different world altogether. The transformation has been in the role of the practice teacher (field instructor), in the recognition of the importance of *theorising from practice* rather than 'putting theory into practice' and the development of a curriculum for learning practice (the *practice curriculum*).

The field is no longer seen as a passive site for the application of theory, whatever that might ever have meant, but as a kind of cauldron that is constantly generating theory. The student's supervisor does not help students 'apply' theories, but draws theory from their experience of practice. So, practice learning and teaching has become recognised as its own method or pedagogy; indeed, it is the 'signature pedagogy' of social work education, a very particular speciality.

A consequence of all this has been the relative equality that practice education has achieved in the curriculum (via the notion of a *practice curriculum*) as a full partner with the academy. This is certainly true in terms of the time spent on placement; as noted, 50 per cent in the UK, and in the US a minimum of 400 hours of field education for Bachelor's programmes and 900 hours for Master's. However, work done on placements still does not usually carry academic credit in the way that other modules do, though this is changing, too.

WHAT STUDENTS DO AND LEARN ON PLACEMENTS

There is a learning agreement negotiated by the university tutor, the student and the placement, giving practical details, expectations and opportunities for learning. Students have 'learning outcomes', which include national standards for social work, and the learning agreement spells out what the student is expected to achieve and how. Placements are, nevertheless, highly individual experiences, varying from site to site, and two students can experience the same placement most differently. Here is an example of a learning outcome:

> The student will identify support networks, access them and work with them. Activities that might aid the student's learning could be to complete a life story with a service user to discover what networks, if any, figure in their history; to meet with a group of service users in a local day care centre to discuss networks with the group; interview local

voluntary group leaders to understand how they provide support in the community and how networks develop and are accessed. Later in the placement, the student might introduce a service user to a support network and take part in an evaluation of how the network functions and what improvements could be made.

Although placements take place in a specific setting (such as a children and families team or a multiprofessional mental health unit) the social work that they are learning transcends the specific setting; so, to take the above example, their learning about support networks is not specific to a particular service user group and it is important for students to consider how they can transfer their learning from this setting and this service user group to others. It is possible to encounter only a fraction of all the possible specific settings for social work, so the skill of transferring learning from one situation to another is absolutely critical.

HOW STUDENTS ARE ASSESSED ON PLACEMENTS

As noted earlier, students cannot achieve a qualification in social work without passing all of their placements. In the event of a fail, in some circumstances the student might be given an extended period or another placement. In addition to proving their competence, students must also show that they are *suitable* for professional practice; professional misconduct can see them removed from the programme.

Most social work programmes base their assessment of students' placement learning around competences (see the discussion earlier). 'Indicators' are developed to break each competence into smaller behavioural units, but there are also approaches, such as the case study, that let the student tell the wider story.

Increasingly, it is social work students themselves who must collect evidence of their competence, assisted in this task by their supervisors. In the UK the evidence is usually gathered in a document called a *portfolio*, often structured around the various occupational standards that the student is expected to achieve. Some portfolios prompt the student to provide a description, an analysis and a subsequent reflection on various aspects of their learning and practice.

In addition, the student's supervisor (known as practice teacher, practice educator or field instructor) writes a report of their assessment of the student, including direct observations of the student with service users. A minimum number of direct observations is specified in the different countries of the UK. The documentation is also likely to include statements and testimonies from service users and colleagues of the student and, in the more creative portfolios, any artefacts that supplement the picture of the student's abilities.

A recommendation is made by the student's practice teacher. A sample of portfolios is reviewed, often by a panel, to ensure that standards are consistent across and between programmes. This process is referred to as moderation. As the university has overall responsibility for the quality of social work education, including the placements, the final decision to accept the recommendation lies with the university's Examination Board.

THE ORGANISATION OF SOCIAL WORK EDUCATION

ACADEMY AND AGENCY PARTNERSHIPS

The quality of a student's experience of social work education relies on a partnership between the class and the field, sometimes referred to as 'academy and agency'. Often informal, this partnership is sometimes formalised, for example via a service contract in which an agency agrees to supply an agreed number of placements over a particular period. A reciprocal agreement might see the university providing seminars for the staff of a partner agency.

Some social workers and managers teach on local programmes, participate in the selection of students and in meetings to adjudicate on a student's conduct. Increasingly, this partnership is becoming three-way, with the involvement of service users in these educational management activities.

FUNDING

Placements are a contribution to the future development of the social work profession and, in most cases, students give as much as they take from the agencies where they are placed. They can be a valuable resource. However, in an attempt to improve the quality of placements, the UK has for some time offered payments to organisations willing to provide student learning. These daily placement fees are a specified amount paid for each day of a student's placement, designed to cover the teaching, the assessment and the administration of the placement. Some smaller agencies in particular have found this fee to be a financial lifeline, but if they are not able to offer quality supervision themselves they must use part of the fee to buy the time of an independent practice teacher to supervise the students. Placement funding in the UK is under review and by no means secure.

The class-based learning is funded in England by direct grants of money from central government via the Higher Education Funding Council for England (HEFCE). These monies are being substantially reduced, with individual students expected to fill the gap with higher tuition fees.

WORKFORCE PLANNING

The numbers of students and placements are such that a person or team is often employed to co-ordinate this work. This Practice Learning Co-ordinator is frequently part of a team working with the broader concerns of recruitment and retention of social workers and the training needs of the wider workforce. The quality of the experience of a placement can affect the recruiting reputation of the agency and have knock-on effects on the morale of the staff overall.

With accurate data, it is possible to predict the likely need for qualified social workers in different regions and, therefore, the numbers of students required to satisfy it. 'Skills councils' in the UK are responsible for co-ordinating this level of planning, not just for social work training but also for the needs of the general social care workforce.

SUPERVISION

Supervision is a key element in the support of social workers and students. Classically, supervision incorporates educational, supportive and administrative (managerial) functions and, more especially with students, also assessment. However, the term 'supervision' is not necessarily self-evident and for people with an industrial background it might be strongly identified with instruction and oversight of their work. It is important, then, to open discussion about mutual expectations of supervision from the beginning of a new supervisory relationship.

STUDENT SUPERVISION AND AGENCY SUPERVISION

Student supervision is more likely to be educative in nature, based on the principles of adult learning discussed earlier. The student's case experiences are used as a prism for the student's learning and the supervisor might use simulations, articles, discussion and the like to accelerate the student's learning. Agency supervision for social work practitioners tends to be more managerial, a 'case of the week' approach with discussion limited to current cases, especially those causing any concerns, and notification of any changes in agency procedures and policies. Sometimes the one kind of supervision leaks into the other; some team leaders who are experienced as student supervisors are keen to make the experience of agency supervision more educational and less inspectorial.

Although supervision is a totem of the social work profession, its quality and frequency varies. In a 2008 poll of 422 UK social care professionals (a wider group than social workers), 28 per cent said they received no supervision and 31 per cent that the supervision was not adequate (*Community Care*, March 2010).

The UK Social Work Reform Board recommends 90 minutes of regular, uninterrupted supervision for all social workers. The stress and complexity of social work is believed to benefit from periods of reflection, to see the wood away from the trees. However, knowledge of what kinds of supervision work best in which kinds of situation is limited and we need more empirical evidence about effective supervision.

INDEPENDENT SUPERVISION

There is an argument that professional supervision should be separated from agency supervision. Social workers need to express their feelings honestly if they are to grow professionally, but this is constrained if the supervisor is also their line manager, a person with hierarchical power. This line of reasoning points towards a model where social workers receive managerial oversight from their agency supervisor and professional development from an independent supervisor. This model is not uncommon in Sweden where independent professional supervision is often provided in small groups. However, decisions have to be made about who meets the additional costs of the independent supervisor – the supervisees, their agency or a combination.

METHODS OF TEACHING STUDENT SOCIAL WORKERS

Supervision for students on placement should be a weekly experience of at least an hour and a half. It is where all the experiences of the preceding week are gathered together and the student is helped to make sense of them. In addition to enhancing the student's learning, the supervisor is ensuring that the student is giving an adequate service to the agency's clients and is also making assessments of the student's abilities.

When the supervisor and the student are together with the service users, this is an opportunity for 'live supervision', with the supervisor guiding the student's practice by direct observation and intervention. It needs to be carefully prepared so that everyone involved is comfortable with the experience, understands its purpose and gives free consent to it.

Some students have the chance to take part in group and peer supervision. Students can learn much from one another, with a group generating more ideas, solutions and challenges than one-to-one, as long as it is facilitated by someone who is experienced with group dynamics. There are many methods of teaching that are transferable between the class and the field setting:

Case discussion, critical incident analysis, reflective diaries, policy analysis, online article searches, graphic techniques with flipcharts, and simulated activities and exercises including role play and rehearsal.

These are all methods to help student social workers to learn about good practice and how to achieve it.

LAW AND SOCIAL WORK

Social work has a very close relationship to law and in some fields of practice, such as mental health, adoption and child protection, a close knowledge of the legal framework is critical, though social workers rely on legal specialists for detailed expertise. Legal underpinning for social work as a profession is also important; in some countries it is listed by government statute as a recognised profession.

Law is, of course, highly specific to nation-states. The amount of law that has a direct impact on social work practice and the extent to which it is enforced varies from country to country and, in federal nations, from state to state. The law sets out principles for practice and for the distribution of resources, supported by government directive and guidance and by the accumulation of case law, i.e. the interpretation of the law in the courts. The law seeks to make concepts clear and unambiguous, but it cannot guarantee good practice. For example, the Mental Capacity Act makes the notion of 'mental capacity' explicit, yet there is evidence from practice that there is often a presumption of incapacity, contrary to the spirit and principles of the Act.

Social work is named in some laws as having specific statutory obligations that can only be discharged by social workers, in some cases involving the removal of liberty from individuals; 'statutory work' also refers to social work that uses legal provisions, whether social work is mentioned specifically or not.

It is important for social workers to keep abreast of changes and proposed changes to the law. In England, for instance, the Law Commission's recommendations for social care legislation specifically mention social work as a community care service, which could help reinforce social work as a method of intervention.

Below is an indication of the legislation that is significant for a social worker who is the manager of an organisation providing social services for and with people with learning disabilities in an English town. It shows the breadth of the relevant legislation in just one setting.

With thanks and acknowledgements to Jackie King-Owen, Chief Executive of *Enable*.

SOCIAL CARE	HEALTH
Registered Care Homes Act 1984	Better Services for Mental Health 1971
Small Homes (Amendment) Act 1991	National Health Service Act 1977
Carers (Recognition/Services) Act 1995	Health Act 1999
Direct Payments Act 1996	Valuing People 2001
Carers and Disabled Children Act 2000	Mental Capacity Act 2005

Care Standards Act 2000

Carers (Equal Opportunities) Act 2004

Valuing People Now 2006

Health Act 2006

Health and Social Services and Social Security Adjudications Act 1983

National Health Service and Community Care Act 1990

Health and Social Care Act 2008

HOUSING

Housing (Homeless Persons) Act 1977

Housing Grants, Construction and

Regeneration Act 1996

Housing Act 1996

GENERAL

Charities Act 2006

Companies Act 1985; 2006

Race Relations Act 1965; 1976; 2000

The Equality Act 2010

DISABILITY MOVEMENT

Mental Health Act 1959

Disabled Persons (Services

Consolidation and Representation) Act 1986

Disability Discrimination Act 1995

Data Protection Act 1998

Human Rights Act 1998

Freedom of Information Act 2000

Mental Capacity Act 2005

OTHER SIGNIFICANT ASPECTS OF THE LAW

Social workers need to know if their employer is not fulfilling its legal obligations and how to take appropriate action, at first within the organisation but if necessary outside it. For instance, in responding to cuts in funding, are proposals to close a day centre legal?

Broader laws are significant to social work, such as human rights legislation and any measures that lessen or deepen poverty; for instance, strategies to reduce child poverty will be obligatory for every local authority in Wales (under provisions of the Children and Families [Wales] Measure, 2010). These and many other acts are not specific to social work but social workers need to be aware of them.

Social work practice is affected by the speed with which the courts act. In 2010 children in the UK were waiting an average 57 weeks in unstable family homes and emergency foster placements before a county court could decide on a more permanent future for them. The figure for 1989 was 12 weeks, so there has been a marked deterioration. One theory to explain this delay is that judges ask for independent assessments (which take time) rather than accepting those of social workers, itself a concern for the profession in terms of its reputation and status. Finally, the costs of the law are significant, and the court fees paid by local authorities for care and supervision proceedings are considerable.

CIVIL DAMAGES

Increasingly, social workers are subject to civil damages, for example in respect of removing children from their families. Social workers were largely immune to claims of negligence, but the situation changed in England with the Human Rights Act 1998. There is a risk that imposing a duty of care on social workers will induce defensive practice that focuses on a desire to prevent possible future legal action rather than the child's needs. Social workers should be able to make judgements without having to consider the threat of litigation; if there have been serious shortcomings these can be dealt with via the conduct panel of the professional body.

AFTER QUALIFICATION

LICENSING AND REGISTRATION

In social work, an academic qualification, such as the degree, is separate from the professional qualification, though the latter cannot be gained without the former. In many countries there is a system of licensure or registration, which protects the title of social worker and restricts the practice of social work to those who are registered.

NEWLY QUALIFIED SOCIAL WORKERS

The role of social workers in their first year after qualification is much debated. Should they be able to 'hit the ground running' as soon as they are qualified, or should the first year be seen as a continuation of their learning, with a workload that is limited?

In terms of what it is realistic to expect student social workers to learn in the three or four years of their degree (or two years for a Master's), the obvious answer is that their first year in practice should be a carefully supervised time of orientation to the particular work of the agency where they are employed. Although half of their course has been in work settings (the placements), these have been in the role of student, which is properly different from being a full-time practitioner.

It is understandable that employers want newly qualified workers to solve the problems of under-staffing and poor retention of experienced staff. However, unrealistic expectations are sometimes placed on the new recruits and blame is attached to the social work training courses when these expectations are dashed. Each generation thinks that this is a new problem, but I remember the same complaints in the 1970s. It is important to emphasise that there are many enlightened employers, not necessarily the noisiest, who recognise the needs of new recruits and nurture them accordingly. My own first year as a qualified social worker in the UK was well supervised and my case-load was protected, important for laying firm foundations for future practice.

In fact, social workers accommodate quite readily to the values and working practices of the agency where they are employed and these local cultures are generally stronger than external loyalties, such as those to the professional code. This reinforces the need for assertive social workers, as discussed earlier in the chapter.

CONTINUING PROFESSIONAL DEVELOPMENT

Social workers develop their professionalism informally through good supervision and the opportunity to reflect on their own practice, and formally in post-qualifying training, which includes courses, day conferences and seminars. Some of these might be 'one-off' events and others can form part of post-qualifying programmes that are assessed and, if the social worker is successful, carry credits towards a post-qualifying award. This is likely to be assessed using a portfolio, as described earlier, with some direct observation of the worker by their manager or a mentor. In England the post-qualifying system consists of a series of specialist, higher specialist and advanced awards in areas such as child protection and mental health. Each specialist award has an element that is associated with teaching practice to others.

It is a big challenge to balance the need to develop professionally against the pressures of day-to-day work. A virtuous circle is achieved when a social worker can use the knowledge derived from their professional development to make better sense of their everyday work practices and thereby gain more control of their work. This in turn gives them more time for continuing professional development, and so the positive cycle continues. Learning how to break into this virtuous circle, and to sustain it, is a great achievement.

IN CONCLUSION

Social work is complex and requires a combination of intellectual, emotional and interpersonal abilities. It is establishing itself as its own discipline, with a growing body of research and doctoral studies. The education of social workers relies on a careful balance of academic and professional training; in the UK half of the learning is based in class settings (the academy) and half in practice settings (the agency). The ways in which social work practice is taught and learned have been radically transformed by the development of the notion of a *practice curriculum* to integrate what is learned in class with what is learned during placements.

FURTHER READING

S. Braye and M. Preston-Shoot, with L.-A. Cull, R. Johns and J. Roche, *Teaching, Learning and Assessment of Law in Social Work Education*, London: SCIE/Policy Press, 2009.
A comprehensive review of good practice in the teaching, learning and assessment of law for social work.

M. Doel, *Social Work Placements*, London: Routledge, 2009.
Using a 'Rough Guide' travel book approach, this book takes readers on a journey through *Socialworkland* to highlight placements as adventures.

P. Hawkins and R. Shohet, *Supervision in the Helping Professions* (3rd edition), Buckingham: Open University, 2006.
An individual, group and organisational approach to supervision across a range of professions. The third edition has broadened the approach from an earlier narrower counselling focus.

I. Shaw, K. Briari-Lawson, J. Orme and R. Ruckdeschel (eds), *The Sage Handbook of Social Work Research*, London: Sage, 2010.
An international and encyclopaedic compendium of social work research, more for reference than for reading from cover to cover.

P. Trevithick, *Social Work Skills* (2nd edition), Buckingham: Open University, 2005.
A classic practice handbook with a comprehensive focus on skills.

SOME RELATED WEBLINKS

www.communitycare.co.uk/social-work-degree-social-care-students is a networking site for student social workers.
www.cswe.org Council on Social Work Education (US).
www.collegeofsocialwork.org/pcf.aspx The Professional Capabilities framework.
www.kcl.ac.uk/sspp/kpi/scwru/pubs/2009/husseinetal2009Variations.pdf has further statistics about UK student social workers.
www.nice.org.uk National Institute for Health and Clinical Excellence.
www.scie.org.uk Social Care Institute for Excellence.

REFERENCES

Community Care (2010), 'Solutions in supervision', 15/4/10: 14.
Guardian Weekend (2010), 'Foster carer's diary – August', 27/11/10: 23.

6

UNIVERSAL OR SPECIFIC
SOCIAL WORK LOCAL AND GLOBAL

This chapter considers whether social work is a universal practice or one that is inevitably locked into time and place. It explores the interplay of local and global.

GENERIC AND SPECIALIST

If you were to land in England in 1980 and happened to find yourself in a social work team, it would most likely describe itself as doing patchwork or 'going local'. The team, comprised solely of social workers and social work assistants, would cover a very specific geographical area – population density in urban areas would allow quite a small patch. The workers describe themselves as *generic*, explaining that they each work with people 'from cradle to grave', young and old and with a variety of problems. If they were asked about a specialism they would probably point to different social workers working with specific neighbourhoods within the patch or perhaps a particular practice, such as groupwork.

Fast forward thirty years to the 2010s and almost all these English social workers describe themselves as specialists and take for granted that these specialisms are based largely around age (children, young people, adults) or mental health. There are sub-specialisms, too, such as child protection work and adoption and fostering within the children and families area. Many of these specialists' job titles are no longer social worker and they are in teams where other members are not social workers.

One of the key issues that faces the specialist social worker of the 2010s is how to integrate work with other services when a family has multiple problems; a household where there is a grandmother with early onset dementia, a father with a personality disorder, a mother with sight loss, a child whose behaviour is causing concern at school and a baby who is failing to thrive. The same problem was faced in the 1960s and the response then (via the Seebohm Report) established the generic social services departments that gave birth to the patch team we visited in 1980. The answer to the dilemma of how to provide a unified service might well be answered differently this time round. What is important is the recognition that the fortunes of generic and specialist social work ebb and flow and that the current high tide of specialist services is possibly on the turn.

GENERIC, GENERALIST AND SPECIALIST

Social work grew by aggregation, as we saw in Chapter 1. To use a territorial analogy, social work gradually brought neighbouring professional territories into a kind of social work federation. The associated term *generic* therefore came to mean a form of practice that spread across all of these specialisms. As such, it laid generic social work open to a charge of 'jack of all trades and master of none', a thinly spread practice that could not hope to achieve depth.

Alongside these developments, the notion of *generalist practice* emerged, especially in the US. In fact, generalist practice has its roots in the broad work of the early Settlements that we visited in the first chapter. It is an irony that social work's first steps were, in fact, coherent and unified and that it was only later that they became splintered into various fields of practice which then needed to be pieced back together.

Generalist practice became associated with basic practice, a foundation for later specialist practice (and, in the US, *advanced* practice). In this hierarchical model of the division of social work labour, specialist practice is only possible after generalist practice has been mastered, so specialist is seen as implicitly senior. In addition, generic and generalist have become confused with one another.

This is both unfortunate and wrong. It is important that these concepts of generic, generalist and specialist are better understood because they hold the key to a more fundamental understanding of what social work is.

Let us first take generalist and specialist. Social workers work with different systems: individual, family, group, organisation and community. Many social workers operate at only one of these levels and are, therefore, specialists in this respect. A generalist is someone who works with some or all of these systems. In this conceptualisation there is no firm line between specialist and generalist, but a continuum that moves between most specialist (working with just one system of practice) and most generalist (working with all systems).

How does this distinction between generalist and specialist shape up in practice? In the case of a young person failing at school and getting into trouble at home and in the community, it is possible to see how interventions could occur at a number of different points:

- one-to-one with the young person;
- work with the family;
- groupwork with the young person and others in similar situations;
- work with the individual school;
- work with the specific neighbourhood;
- work with the school system as a whole;
- work with the legal system; and
- any combination of these systems.

The focus of the work would depend on a combination of the perceived needs, the skills and knowledge of the worker, the way the particular problems at hand are defined, and the context. A sole generalist practitioner would work with many of these systems; or several specialist workers would work with specific levels. All of them would draw on the *generic core* of social work practice knowledge.

Why is this clearer understanding of the notion of a specialism important to the future of the profession? First, social work is vulnerable if it is defined by the professional territory it happens to find itself able to occupy. This way lies the 'Poland phenomenon', whereby the map of social work's territory is drawn and redrawn by much more powerful neighbours and social work is essentially weak and liable to be wiped off the map completely. (Poland has historically been subject to partition by its more powerful neighbours, Prussia/ Germany, Russia and Austria.) Social work must be defined by its generic core, the way it conceptualises the world, not by the number of specialist territories it can occupy for a brief time.

Second, social work's history as an aggregation of related professional groupings makes it prone to disaggregation. The move to specialisms massively increases the potential for a diaspora, weakening rather than strengthening the bonds that hold the social work parts together. Specialist posts frequently obliterate social work from the job title:

> restorative justice development officer, assertive outreach service practitioner, child protection adviser, personalisation development manager.

They require a social work qualification but do not name the posts as social workers. As social work has become more specialised so it has become less visible as a unitary profession. To use the business language described in Chapter 2, its brand is indistinct.

The future of a unified, strong social work profession lies in the achievement of a balance between generalists and specialists and the sound articulation of the generic social work that underpins them both. The uniqueness of social work is the fact that it does not occupy a specific territory in the way that, say, neurology or family law does. It is a holistic practice whose strength comes from the ability to move between different systems and levels to achieve the broadest understanding and impact.

What is different about social work is not the territory it occupies but the way it conceptualises the world: its spread is, literally, global.

SPECIFICS IN SOCIAL WORK

Now that we understand a specialism as skilled practice at one particular system or level of intervention, we can see that what are often described as specialisms are in fact *specifics* of social work practice. Below are some of the specifics that shape the way social work is practised.

FIELD

The social services departments created in the 1970s in the UK were historically unusual as organisations that employed large numbers of social workers, managed by social workers. More often, social workers have found themselves employed in fields where social work is secondary, such as hospitals, schools and courts. In these fields of medical social work, child welfare and juvenile justice, social work is a secondary activity to medicine, education and law. It is from some of these fields of practice, such as psychiatric social work, that social work coalesced into a unitary profession in the middle years of the twentieth century.

SETTING AND SECTOR

Setting is a loose term, generally understood as differentiating field-work, residential and daycare. In the 1960s residential social work was beginning to establish itself as its own profession, with a specific qualification (residential child care officer) and increasing numbers of qualified staff in residential homes. However, the expansion of community-based social work and more attractive salaries were factors that drained qualified staff away from residential to field settings. Attempts to develop an educational 'pathway' solely for residential social work faltered and merged instead with a general child care pathway.

In the UK, the distinctions between sectors is also seen as a specific practice: social work in the statutory (state and governmental), private (for profit) and voluntary (charitable and not for profit) sectors. (See pages 118–20.)

SERVICE USER GROUPINGS

The common way of defining 'specialism' in the UK in the 2010s is by the age of service users; thus, the main organisational distinction is between children's services and adult services. The third major specific is mental health. The result is that social work is a smaller player in mental health services, which are dominated by the National Health Service, and in children's services, merged into the larger education departments. 80 per cent of the new children's department heads have an education rather than a social work background.

It is difficult to know the long-term impact on social work identity. Will social workers in mental health increasingly identify themselves as a 'mental health specialist' rather than a social worker and would that matter? One contributor to an online forum described mental health social workers as having no understanding of child protection: 'They have a similar view of social workers as their clients – that we [child protection workers] are out to get them – and end up advocating for their client and undermining child protection. It happens so often that it's frightening' (CareSpace forum, reported in *Community Care*, 7/4/11: 16). This does not read as one social worker speaking about other social workers.

How do social models of practice fare when the dominant professional model is medical? Those who are strongly committed to these developments point to the benefits of specialised knowledge and working together with other professionals in the team. Its critics suggest that the notion of specialism is itself based on a medical model inherently contradictory to social work as a holistic practice.

The people who use social work do not divide their lives into categories. For example, parental mental health is a significant factor for children entering the care system and children's social workers estimate that well over half of the parents on their caseloads have mental health problems, or misuse alcohol or substances (Office of the Deputy Prime Minister, 2004). There are many young carers of parents with mental health issues. With almost no generalist social work practitioners working across client groups, the balance needs to be redressed.

LOCATION

Every neighbourhood has its own qualities and the biggest distinction is between urban and rural. Attlee, writing in 1920, proposed twinning specific urban and rural neighbourhoods, describing this kind of community activism as social work. In current times the greatest differences between urban and rural settings for social workers are the relative dispersal or concentration of resources and the stability or transience of the populations.

METHOD

Psychosocial casework, systemic family work and gestalt groupwork are all examples of specialist methods for which social workers might have experienced additional training and expertise. Social work methods have become less significant as teaching in this area has declined in the social work curriculum. What might have been a sequence of ten three-hour workshops on groupwork is typically reduced to a day's lecture and seminars. The resurgence of social work methods as a specific social work practice would strengthen the profession's confidence and identity.

EXPERTISE

In the US there is a notion of advanced practice based on expertise. Generalist practice is taught at BSW level (Bachelor's) and Advanced practice at MSW (Master's), thus emphasising the notion of junior and senior practices discussed earlier. The Council on Social Work Education declares that 'BSW [generalist] practice incorporates all of the core competencies' and that 'Advanced practice incorporates all of the core competencies *augmented by knowledge and practice behaviors specific to a concentration.*' 'Augmented' is suitably vague.

Specialist (*specific* according to our definition) social work is enshrined in the post-qualifying education that is available to social workers in England. The demarcation of 'areas of practice' can be seen as ones of expertise:

- children and young people, their families and carers;
- leadership and management;
- practice education;
- social work in mental health services;
- social work with adults.

ORGANISATIONAL FORM

In-take teams work with service users at the first point of contact, usually to complete short-term pieces of work and to decide which situations will be referred to the long-term team of social workers. Out-of-hours emergency teams provide urgent social work services outside the normal hours. These are examples of social work practice that are specific to time.

Social work management might be considered a specific social work practice, though it is seldom considered in this way; rather it is a generic notion of management that prevails, with the implicit message that management skills can be transferred between management roles, social work or otherwise.

Let us move on to consider the specifics that are developing in the different countries of the United Kingdom.

COUNTRIES OF THE UNITED KINGDOM

Social, cultural and legal variations across the four countries of the UK shape social work in diverse ways, accentuated by political devolution. There is some evidence that attitudes to social work might be shaping differently, too. For example, the behaviour of politicians towards social workers following child murders is illuminating. The populist criticism by an English cabinet minister at the time of the 'Baby P' murder in London contrasted to the support for social workers from Scotland's First Minister at the time of a child murder in Dundee. Welsh Assembly ministers have criticised 'outmoded managerialism' and signalled an intention to promote relationship-based work.

Below is a brief review of some of the repercussions for social work of the diverging policies and practice in the four countries.

SOCIAL POLICIES

England, Scotland, Wales and Northern Ireland have developed variations in social policies for some time. An example is the children's hearings system and criminal justice social work in Scotland, which differ from those in the other countries of the UK. Political devolution is accelerating this divergence as decisions about the direction for social services are devolved to all four countries.

Social work is free in all four nations. In Scotland there are no charges for personal care for older people at home nor in care homes. Although there are concerns in some quarters about the cost of this policy, free personal care accounts for less than eight per cent of the £4.5bn spent on health and social care for older people in Scotland. An upper limit on charges for social care is mooted in Wales. Free personal care for all was rejected in Northern Ireland in 2009. In England each council sets its own charges for social care; the main thrust is consumerist with an emphasis on personal budgets.

In Northern Ireland there is a single 'threshold' for judging whether people are eligible to receive social work and social care. England and Wales have four levels by which eligibility is assessed: critical, substantial, moderate or low. In Scotland thresholds vary between councils.

The age of criminal responsibility has been raised from 8 to 12 in Scotland (in line with much of Europe), though it remains at 10 in the rest of the UK. The children's hearing systems in Scotland focus on the children's welfare needs as well as offending. The youth justice system is under review in Northern Ireland. Young offenders appear before youth courts in England and Wales.

There are a number of legislative changes that move social work in Wales further away from that in England, such as a requirement for each local authority to have strategies in place to reduce child poverty and new family support teams that integrate different services. The Welsh language is strong and there is guidance about the way language shapes and alters realities as well as meanings. These ideas have relevance for international social work.

Race is the principle social division in England, and to a lesser extent also in Scotland and Wales, but in Northern Ireland it is sectarianism. Although the Good Friday Agreement and power sharing have led to quieter times, the strong division between Protestant and Catholic communities remains the key fault line for public services like social work.

England is by far the largest of the four nations. With England as 100, the ratios are 100: 10 (Scotland): 6 (Wales): 3.5 (Northern Ireland). The population of Yorkshire, England's largest county, is the same as Scotland's, so it is no surprise that the notion of 'England' conceals huge regional variations and disparities. The social and political demographics of northern England have much more in common with Scotland and Wales than with southern England, and it is likely that a devolved northern England would follow social policies more aligned to those of Scotland and Wales, such as free social care for adults, a national care service and a citizen-focused rather than a consumerist approach.

Our focus on the divergence of the nations should not obscure the similarities between them. Trends in social attitudes, which in themselves influence legislation and social work practice, are often consistent. So, although the decriminalisation of homosexuality occurred at different times (1968 in England and Wales, 1980 in

Scotland and 1981 in Northern Ireland), the growth of social liberalism has been a feature in all four countries in the second half of the twentieth century.

ORGANISATION OF SERVICES

The separation of social work into children's and adult services in England started in the 1990s and during the next decade, education and social work amalgamated into children's departments. Children's and adults' social services do not have quite such a clear separation in Wales, where there are moves to organise social work services regionally, even nationally, rather than locally.

In Scotland, too, local councils have responsibility for social services, but the degree to which adults' and children's services are integrated or separated varies from one authority to another. There is no separate probation service and this work is undertaken by criminal justice social workers, who are part of the local authorities' social work departments. The Scottish government has announced an intention to integrate adult social care and health services. In Northern Ireland a single health and social care board buys services and five local boards are responsible for providing them.

There are a number of test sites in England for a new form of social work organisation based on the social enterprise movement (see pages 120–1).

ORGANISATION OF SOCIAL WORK EDUCATION

More than eighty universities and colleges in England offer social work degree courses, eight in Scotland, eight in Wales and six in Northern Ireland. In Scotland undergraduate courses are mostly four years (full-time), though this may change, and three years in the other countries.

The challenges of social work education outlined in the previous chapter are common to all four countries, not least finding best ways to integrate class-based and agency-based learning and finding placements of good quality. Sometimes the differences are more notable within the countries than between them: for example, the dearth of placements in one area compared to a well-developed system of provision in another. There are particular developments in some countries that are of mutual interest, such as the first National Social Work Student Forum in Wales and the creation of a comprehensive database of placements in Northern Ireland. Local authorities in Wales are committed to providing a specific number of placements when a social work programme is validated. An Assessed Year in Employment following qualification as a social worker has been in place in Northern Ireland since 2006 and is planned for other countries of the UK.

REGULATION

The regulatory bodies register social workers and, in some cases, social work students and some social care staff. They maintain lists of approved social work degree courses. In England the functions of the General Social Care Council (GSCC) transfer, somewhat controversially, to the Health Professions Council (HPC) in 2012. Equivalent bodies are the Scottish Social Services Council (SSSC), the Care Council for Wales (Cyngor Gofal Cymru) and the Northern Ireland Social Care Council (NISCC).

Ofsted regulates children's social services in England and inspects councils' performance in this field. The Care Quality Commission regulates adult services but does not inspect. Scottish children's and adults' services are regulated and inspected by Social Care and Social Work Improvement Scotland; the Welsh equivalent is the Care and Social Services Inspectorate Wales and in Northern Ireland it is the Office of Social Services at the Department of Health, Social Services and Public Safety. The Care Standards Act (2000) still stands in Wales but has been replaced by the Health and Social Care Act (2008) in England, creating a new regulatory system.

Differences in the local context are likely to make cross-country movement within the UK increasingly difficult.

INTERNATIONAL SOCIAL WORK

This section unpicks what is universal and what is specific about social work across countries and continents, and the cross-border problems that are the concerns of social work. We will consider the impact of globalisation on social work.

SOCIAL WORK'S INTERNATIONAL PRESENCE

Curiosity about social work practices across national borders was in evidence as far back as the 1880s, when American social worker Jane Addams worked with German social worker Alice Salomon to initiate international social work associations, including the Women's International League for Peace and Freedom. Since then, social work's presence has grown around the world, though – in terms of numbers – this presence varies considerably.

One survey, limited to European countries, reported a variation from one social worker per 50 inhabitants in Sweden to one for 2,730 in Germany (reported in *Community Care*, 9/9/10: 9, based on International Federation of Social Workers figures). This seems hardly credible, but it does draw our attention to the difficulty of gathering this kind of basic data and knowing who to count as a social worker and what counts as social work.

If a comparison between two neighbouring European countries is problematic, it is an even greater challenge to estimate the inhabitants per social worker in India or China or Chad. The idea of 'social worker' is much more fluid than, say, doctor or teacher, and many countries do not have the infrastructure to employ social workers in the state apparatus or to gather numbers about their employment elsewhere. For example, in transcaucasian Georgia, there were fewer than ten qualified social workers in 2005 (all of whom were Georgians trained in the US) and the first qualifying courses were not established until 2006. Even so, much of the activity that we recognise as social work was being undertaken, for better or worse, by unqualified Georgian workers.

WHAT IS INTERNATIONAL SOCIAL WORK?

Many social workers are involved in cross-cultural work within one community, some in transnational work across nations, and others are working in countries that are foreign to them. At these very basic levels, social work has become international. However, there are other, subtler interpretations of the meaning of 'international social work'. Indeed, 'international' as an idea is surprisingly complicated. Whereas inter*professional* means work involving at least two professions, the meaning of international is not confined to work involving at least two nations. For instance, in the assessment of the quality of research in British universities, 'international' was used to denote research of exceptional quality that had significance beyond the UK, even if that research was confined just to one nation.

In what ways, then, can social work be construed as international? First, there is a fundamental and universal commitment to challenge injustice that transcends location. Second, physical and intellectual contact across borders is promoted through international associations, exchange programmes and journals of social work. Third, there has been a steady internationalisation of social problems with the result that social workers work locally with people who in various ways are influenced by international events; and lastly, social work plays a part in the international response to world events, with social workers employed by international organisations. International social work refers, then, to a particular *perspective* on practice.

Less well developed is the idea that a social work background, with its holistic approach and its combination of the interpersonal, the organisational and the political, is an excellent grounding for leading international problem-solving teams. A social worker who can negotiate the no-man's land of some neighbourhood estates, and bring about dialogue between people at the margins of society and the mainstream, is someone with much to offer conflict resolution on the international stage.

The ideologies of the liberal democracies (the West or sometimes the Global North) have a dominance in intellectual, cultural and social ideas. Social work is embedded in this ideology, as we discovered in the first chapter. It is ironic, then, that it is in these countries of the West that social work finds itself in some crisis, at odds with the prevailing values of liberal economics and the dominance of the market as the definer of social relations. For this reason it is not easy to predict what social work paradigm might prevail internationally in, say, two or more decades' time.

However, a word of caution about the so-named Western paradigm. It is often presented uncritically as though 'the West' were a homogeneous conglomerate, wholly identified with notions of individualism and economic liberalism. This dishonours the very strong radical movements in the West that emphasise collectivity and community solidarity, especially amongst labour and women's movements, which gave birth to the welfare state. 'The West' has many identities.

LOCAL CONTEXT

It will be clear at this point in the book how social work is shaped by the local context. This is true to some extent of all professions and vocations, but the central importance in social work of untangling social meanings and working with social policies makes it a particularly context-bound activity. Let us illustrate this with the idea of 'mental illness'.

> Over time and place, the behaviours that we associate with mental illness have variously been described as mad, creative, eccentric, evil, feeble minded, magical, wise, anti-social, and the list continues. To some it is a disorder of the psyche, to others a spiritual state, an existential crisis, a neural malfunction or a mutant chromosome, and to others a social phenomenon or learned behaviour. The causes and meanings of 'mental illness', and therefore the response it requires or respects, are almost wholly culturally determined.

We expect there to be differences in the way unusual behaviours are explained in tribal Congo and in urban Britain, but there can be a chasm of difference between neighbours in the same community:

> In my own small patch I had one family explain the condition of their son, diagnosed as mentally ill, as the work of the devil; whilst another family in a nearby street were happy to take a medical diagnosis of schizophrenia to explain their son's behaviour. Social workers are part of this context, too. They bring their beliefs and backgrounds to their work, at times chiming with the service users and at other times not. So, I explained that, though I did not have a personal belief that there was a devil, I did want to find out more about their beliefs and how this affected our approach to their son's situation. (I was sceptical of the idea of 'schizophrenia' as a condition, too.)

Beliefs are all-powerful, so it is important to respect them, but we can do this without sharing them: 'starting where the client is' without having to *be* where the client is.

GLOBAL CONTEXT

People must be understood in their local context, but they can be helped and supported more effectively by social workers who are aware of the global background and who know how the one has an impact on the other.

The increasingly free movement of money and people has given greater power to global capital and has had a large impact on migration as well as weakening the power of local labour. A social worker working in a community where the local large employer has closed because the work has been outsourced to cheaper labour in China will face a community not just with rising levels of unemployment, but also higher rates of mental ill-health, crime and drug and alcohol dependency. Tour the ex-pit villages of South Yorkshire to witness how devastating the effects are and how long they last.

The free movement of information has internationalised knowledge. Virtual communities can use the new technologies of social networks in ways that were unimaginable not long ago; if these had been available during the UK miners' strike in 1984–85, one can imagine a quite different outcome. On the other hand, the ownership of influential media by individual plutocrats keen to preserve their own privileges threatens the value base of social work – collectivism, redistribution of social and economic wealth, social and economic justice and empowering, inclusive social policies. Ideas that were taken for granted, such as the state's role in the redistribution of wealth and the regulation of capital, are challenged, and inequalities have steadily risen. These trends are global and they present social work with increasing workloads as the social infrastructure is weakened and collectivist solutions decline. As the power of the state recedes, must social work also decline? We will consider the further effects of globalisation in the last chapter.

GLOBAL TOPICS

The International Federation of Social Workers has had representative status with the United Nations since 1964 to act in consultative and advocacy roles. These are the kinds of issue that it might advise on:

- people trafficking, slavery (illegal and forced movement of people as commodities) and people smuggling (illegal movement with consent);
- asylum seekers;
- working with street children;
- violence against women;
- refugees;
- homelessness;
- mental health issues;
- HIV/AIDS;
- comparative social work;
- drug trade and alcohol misuse;
- deinstitutionalisation;
- rehabilitation of child soldiers;
- poverty, politics and corruption.

These topics were identified in an international survey of social work students studying international social work.

Migration of peoples, whether it is forced or with a degree of choice, is probably the most significant area of work for social work. Migration is a timeless phenomenon and the UK is a country with a long history of emigration and immigration: five and a half million British people (almost a tenth) live outside the UK and 7.5 per cent of the UK population were born abroad.

People move for many different reasons, primarily economic or political, and the degree to which this movement is voluntary or enforced varies. Forced migration can take place within one country, such as the internally displaced persons (IDPs) in Georgia following the civil wars in the 1990s.

Migration of *ideas* in social work is less well charted. Family Group Conferencing is an example of the transferability of methods from lay communities to professional and, in this case, from the Maori to the Western community. I was taught an American-derived social work method, localised for the UK, then adapted as an educational model for social work students, which I then taught to Russian colleagues, who subsequently visited the UK to teach a variant to English social workers. There are no doubt many such migrations of ideas and practices, usually not tracked, contributing to social work's mixed heritage.

On World Social Work Day in 2011 (15 March), the International Federation of Social Workers (IFSW) called on all social workers to:

- ensure nations meet the most basic human rights to food and shelter, clothing and medical care for all their people;
- raise awareness about poverty as a human rights violation in all countries;
- implement the IFSW policy on poverty eradication;
- champion the Social Protection Floor Initiative of the UN, which ensures universal social protection to health, education, shelter and security, as pledged in the Universal Declaration of Human Rights;
- demonstrate improvements in people's lives.

These broad aspirations need action plans, so it would be interesting to speculate what it would be most appropriate to *do* to celebrate each year's World Social Work Day.

SIMILARITIES

We have considered a wide variety of different interpretations of international social work, the significance of the local context in shaping social services and the wisdom of understanding how the local connects with the global. We must make sure, though, that the emphasis on the differences does not obscure what is common to social work, whether it is practised here or there. The International Federation of Social Workers describes the common values of social work wherever it is practised:

> Social work grew out of humanitarian and democratic ideals, and its values are based on respect for the equality, worth and dignity of all people. Since its beginnings over a century ago, social work practice has focused on meeting human needs and developing human potential. Human rights and social justice serve as the motivation and justification for social work action. In solidarity with those who are disadvantaged, the profession strives to alleviate poverty and to liberate vulnerable and oppressed people in order to promote social inclusion.
>
> (IFSW, 2000)

COMPARATIVE PRACTICE

The role of the state, informal care, ideas of family and childhood, the demographics of a country and, of course, the human and physical resources of a nation are each of huge significance in shaping the local expression of social work. For example, the median age of a population (which varies from 43 years in Japan to under 15 years in Uganda) has enormous implications for social policy and local social work practices.

The notion of the family and, in particular, the role of women in families and in the workforce influences the shape of social work and offers opportunities for comparison. Most Western societies accept a variety of family forms, such as one parent or two parents of the same gender, in ways that remain unacceptable in many other societies. These social changes have had their impact on the social work role: now not so much helping with marital and child-rearing problems, but more supporting lone parents or assisting scattered families to connect. Migration frequently leads to conflicts as the norms of one society (such as arranged marriages) rub against the norms of another (love matches), with social workers working in the cross-fire of opposing values.

The idea of the state as the benevolent provider of social welfare is far from common. Indeed, it has really only become an established norm in countries of northern and western Europe, exported to some others, like New Zealand and Canada. The welfare state is less a function of wealth (Britain created its welfare state at a time of extraordinary austerity) and more one of political will and cultural values. Other political systems, such as the Soviet, developed a strong web of social support, but without the intellectual freedoms and cultural pluralism that characterise the Western welfare state. However, the return of unregulated capitalism has been accompanied by sustained attacks on the value of the welfare state and these have changed the way the state's role is cast: less of the direct benevolent provider and more of a manager to plan, set targets and squeeze 'best value' out of the workforce.

In countries where the state has not been seen as benign and where localism has been strong, such as Germany, provision of social services has been shaped by private bodies and by the church. Also, in the reconstruction of Germany following the Second World War,

American preferences for private and voluntary provision held sway. A UK focus on identifying risk – for instance, of child neglect and abuse – through universal services across the whole population contrasts with the US, where access to services is determined by insurance eligibility and limited government funded services.

Although the contrasts to be drawn from international comparisons are the most obvious, a job exchange with a neighbouring team might also provide a surprisingly striking contrast. I described on page 108 the huge differences in practice between two neighbouring social work teams, the contrast being all the sharper because the local demographics were the same. Conversely, work abroad can teach us about similarities. My first job as a qualified social worker was in a large American city and though I experienced different organisational and social cultures, I learned much more about the commonalities of human life beneath the superficial exotic differences. Notions of social solidarity, personal resilience, group support, peer pressure, status, power and authority – these might find different kinds of expression in different communities, but they are universal if we choose to look for them.

International social work emphasises the interdependence between nations, as well as between individuals and their communities within any one society.

CULTURAL COMPETENCE

The most significant border that social workers cross is the border of their own biography. Social workers must transcend their own backgrounds. Historically in the UK, it was the middle classes working in Settlements, but this has changed, so it is just as likely to be a young black working-class social worker working 'across the borders' with white, middle-class adopters.

Because the notion of the relationship is so central, social workers must have the ability to move beyond their own experience and personal biography to understand the meanings that others attach to their lives. For instance, though a family's inability to care for its own child is not unique to one country at one time, the *meanings* attached to this situation do vary, most likely along the continuum from social acceptance to social stigma. Acceptable solutions will also differ: relying on the immediate family or the wider community; or state intervention via resources to support the family; or sanctioning adoption by other families.

Societies and the families within any particular society view notions of shame in their own way. How usual is it to speak about personal matters outside the family? Whereas talk therapy might be a regular feature of Californian society, some Chinese cultures would view family problems as shameful and something not to be revealed to others. A written agreement used by a social worker might be seen as a helpful aide-memoire by some families, but officious and suspiciously legalistic in some Indian cultures.

A social worker can never learn all the possible cultural permutations and this would be a pointless exercise. Cultural competence is not akin to learning a lot of different languages, it is about knowing how to read social situations.

WORKING THROUGH INTERPRETERS

Sometimes social worker and service user might not speak the same language and interpretation is needed. It is too easy to rely on a bilingual family member or neighbour because they happen to be available, and social workers must think carefully about confidentiality and the power relations between the service user and the informal interpreter.

It is better practice to find out whether an interpreter will be needed and to arrange for a trained, independent interpreter. When there is regular work with a particular community a working relationship can be developed with the interpreter and expectations and issues of privacy discussed. The social worker should speak directly to the service user ('I would like to ask you … ') and not with the interpreter ('can you ask her … '). Similarly, the interpreter needs to give responses in the first person from the service user. Part of the value of the interpreter might be their deeper understanding of the particular culture and not just their linguistic ability. It is important for workers and interpreters to keep a check on the level and value of any *social* interpretation. There might be considerable social differences (region, class, gender, age, religion, etc.) between service user and interpreter that make the latter not expecially well qualified to go beyond a strict linguistic interpretation of what is being said. This gap is the more difficult to bridge when using an interpreter with children.

INTERNATIONAL MOBILITY

Social workers migrate and social work students and educators have increasing opportunities for exchange and mobility, as we will explore briefly in this section.

CROSS-NATIONAL ACTIVITIES

International Social Services was established in 1924 in Geneva and it continues to facilitate liaison between social workers around transnational work such as the overseas placement of children. Children and Families Across Borders, a UK organisation, estimates that in any one year about one in a hundred British social workers travels overseas as part of their work, generally to carry out child and family assessments. However, they may well be acting illegally and it is considered better practice to work through local social services, who are more likely to know the cultural and legal context.

International non-governmental organisations (INGOs) such as Save the Children (established following the First World War), The Red Cross (formed in 1863), Red Crescent, Unicef and Caritas, provide transnational services and employment for social workers across the world.

RECRUITMENT FROM OVERSEAS

The UK is popular with foreign social workers, with 6,700 overseas social workers registered with the General Social Care Council in 2011. Continental Europe accounted for about 1,700 (Germany, Romania and Poland the first three), over 1,300 from Australia, nearly 1,150 from South Africa, just over 1,100 from the US and over 900 from India. It is important that overseas recruitment is well planned and mutual expectations are discussed beforehand. A mentor or buddy is a good idea. Styles of feedback for supervision might be quite different, too, with some cultures very direct and others finely nuanced.

Recruiting overseas workers is not a value-free activity. From one side it is under attack from populist politicians pandering to xenophobia, with the result that caps on immigrant numbers lead to staff shortages in many care homes. 17 per cent of people recruited to the UK social care workforce in 2009 came from overseas and in London 57 per cent of all care workers are not British. On the other side of the argument, there are ethical concerns about rich countries poaching people who are needed all the more in their own countries.

WORKING OVERSEAS

Some people find their way into social work via experience of working abroad, such as Voluntary Service Overseas (VSO). There are no figures for the numbers of UK social workers leaving to work overseas, but anecdotally the UK is still as much a country of emigration as immigration. Motivations vary from the pull of an exciting adventure and a hope that the work–life balance will improve, to the push of increasingly bureaucratised work at home and the spectre of cuts and declining resources with which to work.

Social work's reliance on nuanced communication means that most British social workers leave for English-speaking countries, where language is not a barrier. Competition is less intense where there are shortages in skilled occupations, such as child protection social work in Australia.

STUDY EXCHANGES

European Union social work students and educators can use EU funding to arrange exchanges. Erasmus, Socrates and Tempus schemes enable teaching and learning and in some cases research in social work to take place across the EU and with countries in the broader region, such as North Africa, eastern Europe and central Asia. A European PhD network, TiSSA (The International Social Work and Society Academy), holds annual conferences for PhD social work students across the continent.

Social work students are able to enjoy a wide range of placements overseas. Careful planning is needed to ensure their success and, particularly with UK students placed abroad, that they are not disadvantaged because of the tight scheduling of the social work curriculum at home. Other nations are often able to be more flexible. Also, the limited linguistic skills of most British students means that their options are constrained compared to students coming to the UK, whose command of English is usually good.

IN CONCLUSION

How well *does* social work travel, then? Is it a highly contextualised activity that cannot be separated from its time and place or is it a universal set of principles and practices, with key elements that cross borders and endure through time? As the reader will have gathered, despite the dualism in each of the chapter titles in this book, the answer is always 'both'.

Social work's identity is changed as soon as it crosses borders; indeed, as we have seen, it changes from one community to another and within communities. So, in the development of social work education in eastern Europe in the post-Soviet period, it has been really important that the technical assistance provided by Western social workers has avoided the imposition of their own models of social work.

Though the chameleon changes its colour according to its environment, it does remain a chameleon. Social work's constant adaptation to local conditions is, ironically, one of its enduring characteristics. It has universal core values of social justice to combat oppression and poverty. Social work's holistic practice, working with the personal and the political, with individuals in their families in their communities and in their societies, is a constant. It is in need of refreshment in some parts of the globe and very much alive and well in others.

FURTHER READING

S. Banks and K. Nøhr (eds), *Practising Social Work Ethics Around the World: Cases and Commentaries*, Abingdon: Routledge, 2012.
26 cases of ethical dilemma in social work from 22 different countries. A fascinating testimony to both the universal and the specific in social work, with interesting commentaries on the cases from outsiders.

M. Lavalette and I. Ferguson (eds), *International Social Work and the Radical Tradition*, Birmingham: Venture Press, 2010.
Encourages readers to make connections between social work practice and wider social movements through a series of case studies from several different countries including India, Peru, Nicaragua, South Africa and Palestine.

S. Lawrence, K. Lyons, G. Simpson and N. Huegler (eds), *Introducing International Social Work* (Transforming Social Work Practice series), Exeter: Learning Matters/Sage, 2009.

A good all-round introduction to international social work. There are specific chapters relating to children, young people and families, people with mental health issues, international aspects of social work with older people and people with disabilities. The authors work on the idea that 'the global is local is global' to emphasise the interplay between them.

E.R. Tolson, W.J. Reid and C. Garvin, *Generalist Practice: A Task-centered Approach*, New York: Columbia University Press, 1994.

The book provides a thorough background to generalist practice in the American context.

C. Williams, *Social Policy for Social Welfare Practice in a Devolved Wales* (2nd edition), Birmingham: Venture Press, 2011.

Considers social service delivery under political devolution.

The journal *International Social Work* was established in 1957 and is jointly administered by the International Council on Social Welfare, the International Association of Schools of Social Work and the International Federation of Social Workers. It is an English-language journal with abstracts of articles in French, Spanish, Arabic, Chinese and Russian.

SOME RELATED WEBLINKS

www.ccwales.org.uk Care Council for Wales.
www.cfab.uk.net Children and Families Across Borders.
www.cqc.org.uk Care Quality Commission.
www.cssiw.org.uk Care and Social Services Inspectorate Wales.
www.dhsspsni.gov.uk The Office of Social Services at the Department of Health, Social Services and Public Safety.
www.gscc.org.uk General Social Care Council.
www.hpc-uk.org Health Professions Council.
www.iassw-aiets.org International Association of Schools of Social Work.
www.ifsw.org International Federation of Social Workers.
www.iss-ssi.org International Social Services.
www.isw.sagepub.com *International Social Work* journal (six issues a year).
www.niscc.info Northern Ireland Social Care Council.
www.scswis.com Social Care and Social Work Improvement Scotland.
www.socwork.net/sws *Social Work and Society* international online journal.
www.sssc.uk.com Scottish Social Services Council.
www.tissa.net The International Social Work and Society Academy (TiSSA).

REFERENCES

Community Care (2011), 'Never the twain shall meet?', CareSpace forum 7/4/11: 16.

McGregor, K. 'Scotland better served by social workers than England', *Community Care*, 9/9/10: 9.

7

PAST AND FUTURE

THE PIONEERS OF TODAY ARE THE PROPHETS OF TOMORROW (Attlee)

Social work has a long tradition as an activity appealing to notions and feelings of common humanity, both as philanthropy and as radical social change. However, it has a relatively short history as an established profession and an academic discipline. The current manifestation of social work, certainly in societies that are considered to be social democracies, has been shaped by the welfare bureaucracies that employ social workers in large numbers. In developing countries social work remains a largely informal activity, often associated with broader social and political movements. In developed countries without a strong welfare tradition, such as the United States, it is more individualised, a clinical practice with restricted access. Although all professions are shaped by time and place, perhaps none is quite as susceptible as social work.

CHALLENGES

The public scrutiny of social work witnessed in recent years is likely to intensify rather than weaken. This is a challenge for the profession and requires a robust and transparent response, an active and very public discussion of the tensions and dilemmas that social workers face. This is necessary to develop a wider and better understanding of what it is reasonable to expect social work to accomplish. There needs to be a realignment of the balance between the community's responsibilities (to protect its children, for instance) and the obligations of paid professionals. Presently there is an unhealthy dumping of responsibility, in the form of blame, on individual practitioners. Of course, this kind of rebalancing is reliant on broader social and political action to engage individuals and communities in life beyond the front doorstep.

Social workers must challenge the prevailing culture in many of the organisations where they are employed, a culture that is increasingly rule-bound and focused on self-protection. Though professional discretion must always be tempered by fairness and accountability, in order to avoid abuse of professional power, the weight of procedure is in danger of crushing creative social work practice. Service users need to feel confident that their social workers are assertive and can act according to their professional judgement; and the profession needs to attract and retain self-motivating practitioners whose dedication will pay back the respect that they are accorded.

GLOBALISATION

'McDonaldisation' refers to the global influence of Western (and more particularly American) culture, based largely on a business model where the emphasis is on efficiency to maximise profit; a world that offers no surprises and smoothes out local differences. This is significant for social work at a philosophical level, because it runs contrary to the communitarian ethos of social work and its celebration of diversity.

If social work is to play a part in resisting the business model it needs to ally with wider social movements, which means being *partisan*. In fact, this would not be a new development but rather a rebirth of Attlee's 1920 notion of the social worker as an agitator. On this view, social work cannot stand by as a mediator or arbiter in global affairs, but must take a partisan stance to defend humanitarian and progressive policies locally and globally. The current challenge is remarkably similar to the one facing the early social work pioneers described at the beginning of this book.

When the state demonstrated its commitment to social services by funding them it made sense for social workers to work with the state towards a progressive future. This situation has changed. The state is barely able or willing to collect tax from the most wealthy multinationals and relies heavily on the public sector workforce for a regular tax take. Recent decades have witnessed a massive widening of the gap between rich and poor, quite contrary to the basic principles of social work. In these changed circumstances, social work faces a similar decision to that faced by its forerunners: does it stay as a partner of the state and try to reform it from within, or does it take a more radical path outside the state? In some countries with poorly developed state services the latter path is less of a choice and more of a necessity. In countries like the UK with a strong tradition of state provision it would be a step into a relative unknown. Some claim social work enterprises as the radical alternative (see page 120), but there are dangers that these small enterprises will fall prey to big business once they have proved themselves to be desirable and capable of squeezing a profit. It is not easy, then, to decide who are today's pioneers and whether they will be tomorrow's prophets.

AN IDEAL SOCIAL WORK?

In the first chapter I aimed to introduce social work by relating what it is to what it has been, its past to its present. Those major themes have reverberated through subsequent chapters. In these final paragraphs I would like to take stock and consider what social work will be, or rather what I see that it could be, its future. What follows is a very personal take on an ideal social work and, as such, a risky enterprise; for some it might seem more dystopia than utopia. In contrast to the convention of objectivity – never completely attainable, of course – the following is a personal vision for social work.

First, I see social work based in social service centres that serve communities roughly the size, in England, of a political ward, or a collection of villages in rural areas. Some social service centres are part of a health practice, others not. The buildings are attractive without being ostentatious and located on convenient bus routes, with public transport receiving a subsidy. The centre is open evenings and weekends, busy with groups and community activities.

The team is composed of qualified social workers, assistants, administrative staff and a thriving volunteer group. Its diversity reflects the local community and the broader society. The team is composed of generalist and specialist social workers in roughly equal numbers, all working together in the single team based at the centre (see Chapter 6 for more discussion about generalists and specialists).

The service is a universal one. There is no stigma attached to walking through its doors. Most of the team's time is devoted to people who are the most disadvantaged, but the team works to be as inclusive as possible. There is no notion of 'tiers' of service users or 'levels' of work. A number of part-time staff are drawn from the local community as support staff for particular client groups; they are close to them in experience and have a small budget to use as they see fit.

The National Social Service, like the National Health Service, is funded through general taxation and free at the point of delivery. Unlike doctors' health practices, the funding for these 'social practices' is channelled through local government because local democratic accountability is prized. The centres are public bodies and cannot be 'owned'. Each centre runs democratically; service user and community representatives have elected positions on a social service council. The team leader is elected, like the Dean in some university faculties, for a maximum period, perhaps four years.

The day-to-day work of each centre is overseen by its own elected social service council and each centre is regulated in the manner of the external examining systems in universities – by its peers and independently. So, a social worker who has additional regulatory training and is based in a distant social service centre with no other formal links makes an annual inspection of the work of the centre using an agreed protocol.

A central social work team covers all the social service centres in the town, city or county. It is a small team and its role is to service and advise, not manage, the local social service centres. Most important of all, the local teams experience the central team as having backbone. It provides support when the going gets tough and does not buckle to political or media pressure when individual social workers have made the best professional judgement available at the time; and it takes firm action when irregularities or poor practices are exposed. The council employs a Chief Social Worker, who is a qualified, highly experienced social worker not long out of practice with direct access to the chief executive and who writes an annual report on social work for the council.

Decision-making is highly devolved, but there are some services provided centrally by the local authority; for example, a social work team has an idea for a new development that requires an IT solution. They request the services of the central IT team to adapt an aspect of the information system to meet their specifications. There is no 'internal market'; i.e. these services are not costed and charged separately to the social service centre.

Each centre has a research officer; sometimes a dedicated post, at other times a role that is shared amongst those social workers with research training. Information is systematically gathered for the local community's use and to help develop professional practice. Information is aggregated and analysed for its impact on social policy. The data provides material for active lobbying. There is regular engagement with local and sometimes national media. Individual workers are members of 'communities of practice', many of which have international membership, and the team meets regularly to exchange information and discuss learning from their membership of these communities.

Joint appointments with local social work university departments are common. At any one time, it is likely that one member of the team is on exchange with a social worker either in another UK social service centre or overseas, so the team also benefits from the presence of the exchange partner. This results in constant connections with other social work practices and cross-fertilisation of ideas and practices. There is a regular commitment to providing a placement for two students at any one time and MSW (Master's) students are regularly commissioned by the team: for example, to conduct social surveys and to follow through on ideas for short-term research and evaluation projects.

Some centres have developed a reputation for their expertise in particular social work practice methods and students choose to have placements with them on the basis of this. Neighbouring centres conduct comparative research to develop the knowledge and evidence base about which circumstances seem most favourable to which methods, and local university social work staff are commissioned to help build the practice knowledge base. Co-authored papers are submitted regularly for publication.

People who use the centres find them open, accessible and friendly. The local community knows the workers and many will have been into the centre for other reasons (currently there are photographs on the walls in the centre taken at a recent Community Festival). The team has a reputation for responding quickly, so most of its work is preventative rather than driven by crises. When things do occasionally turn nasty there is a large community of professionals and support staff to intervene and provide a firm, supportive and immediate response.

> ... Life in the ideal social work is not as consensually cosy as this utopia implies. The social service council regularly flexes its democratic muscle and there are conflicts between the priorities of the professional and lay team and the council.

The reader might conclude that I have departed far from the 'firm footed realist' in the quotation that opened the first chapter. Yet I have personal experience of almost all of the elements mentioned above, including the subsidised public transport system. Admittedly they were not all at the same time nor in the same place, but there is no logical reason why this should not be. The firm-footed realist might also object to the cost of this ideal social work, yet a National Social Service could be met by a standard rate of taxation at 33 per cent rising above 90 per cent for the very highest salaries. In other words, precisely where they stood when I received my first social work pay cheque. Perhaps utopia is only a couple of mindsets away?

Can an ideal social work system be divorced from an ideal community? In Western countries social work grew out of an industrialised, urban environment and it is tempting, therefore, to have the 'template community' as one that is densely populated, walkable, diverse and, if there are to be richer and poorer, at least they live in close proximity. My first job as a social worker (unqualified) was in a rural county area and I know the additional challenges that come with scarce resources separated by a large landscape devoid of public transport, but also some of the advantages of close-knit rural life.

Having briefly visited a world of what might be, it is important to note that in the world that is, a large survey of social workers in the UK in 2010 found that a majority were positive about becoming and remaining social workers; this despite the size of workloads, the demands of targets, cuts in spending and the like. In addition to feeling that they were making a difference to people's lives, they felt their working environment was aligned to their core beliefs and values. 'I wake up each morning for work with excitement for the day ahead because every day is completely different from the last' (a social worker quoted in *Community Care*, 22/7/10: 15).

... One last return to the social service centre in the ideal social work world. As we leave the centre we pass a man who rattles a bucket. He's collecting. Not for the local hospice or children's ward, because these are now properly funded by the public purse. The banks, however, are facing hard times and must rely on your charity.

REFERENCE

Bailey, S. (social worker) quoted in Lombard D. 'The day the MP called', *Community Care*, 22/7/10: 15.

INDEX OF NAMES

INDEX OF SUBJECTS